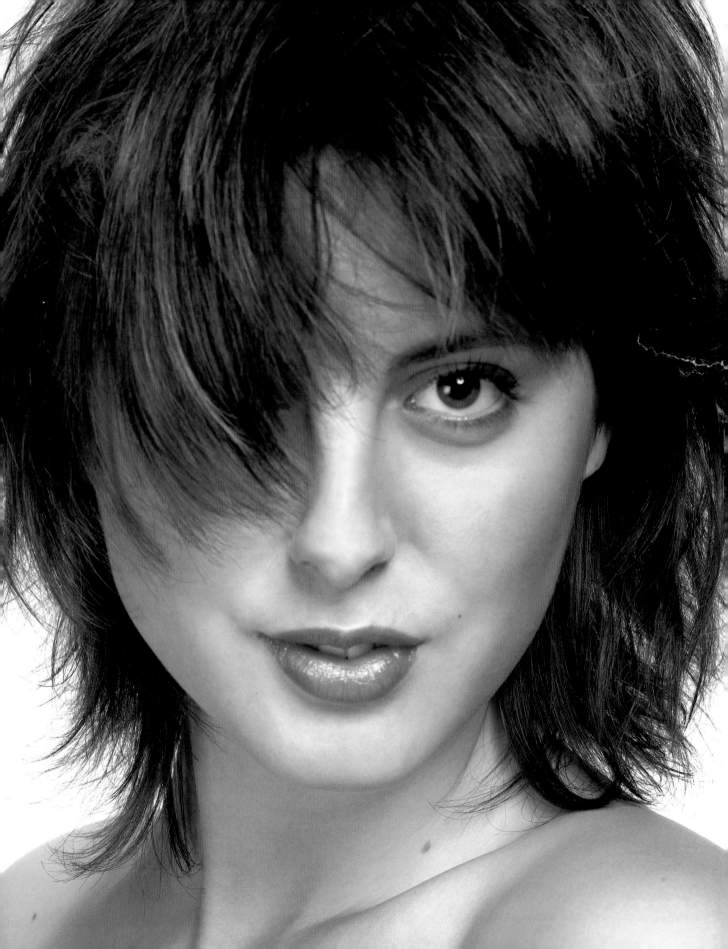

Vincent Roppatte and Sherry Suib Cohen

Cool Hair

A Teenager's Guide to the Best Beauty Secrets on Hair, Makeup, and Style

Photographs by Alex Cao

Illustrations by Wendy DeFeudis

Foreword by Sarah Hughes

St. Martin's Press ❧ New York

www.stmartins.com

Book design by Ralph L. Fowler

Photographs © 2003 by Alex Cao
Illustrations © 2003 by Wendy DeFeudis

Library of Congress Cataloging-in-Publication Data
Roppatte, Vincent.
    Cool hair: a teenager's guide to the best beauty secrets on hair, makeup, and style / Vincent Roppatte and Sherry Suib Cohen; foreword by Sarah Hughes; photographs by Alex Cao; illustrations by Wendy DeFeudis.
        p. cm.
    ISBN 0-312-31251-2
    1. Hairdressing. 2. Hairstyles. 3. Beauty, Personal. 4. Grooming for girls. 5. Teenage girls—Health and hygiene. I. Cohen, Sherry Suib. II. Title.

TT972.R67 2003
646.4'046—dc21   2003046881

First Edition: November 2003

10 9 8 7 6 5 4 3 2 1

I fell in love with my courageous and beautiful wife, Frances,

when we were both teenagers. She taught me every

life lesson I need to know, and this book is

dedicated to her shining memory.

—Vincent Roppatte

Contents

Foreword by Sarah Hughes   xi

1   You're the Best   1

2   Inside Out   13

3   Such Beautiful Hair: Texture and Care   17

4   Cut and Color   41

5   The Elements of Style   63

6   An Adventure: The New You   73

7   Special Occasion Hair   87

8   Get a Grip   109

9   Radiant Skin   113

10   Amazing Face   127

11   Dear Vincent   143

Epilogue   151

Resources   155

Acknowledgments   157

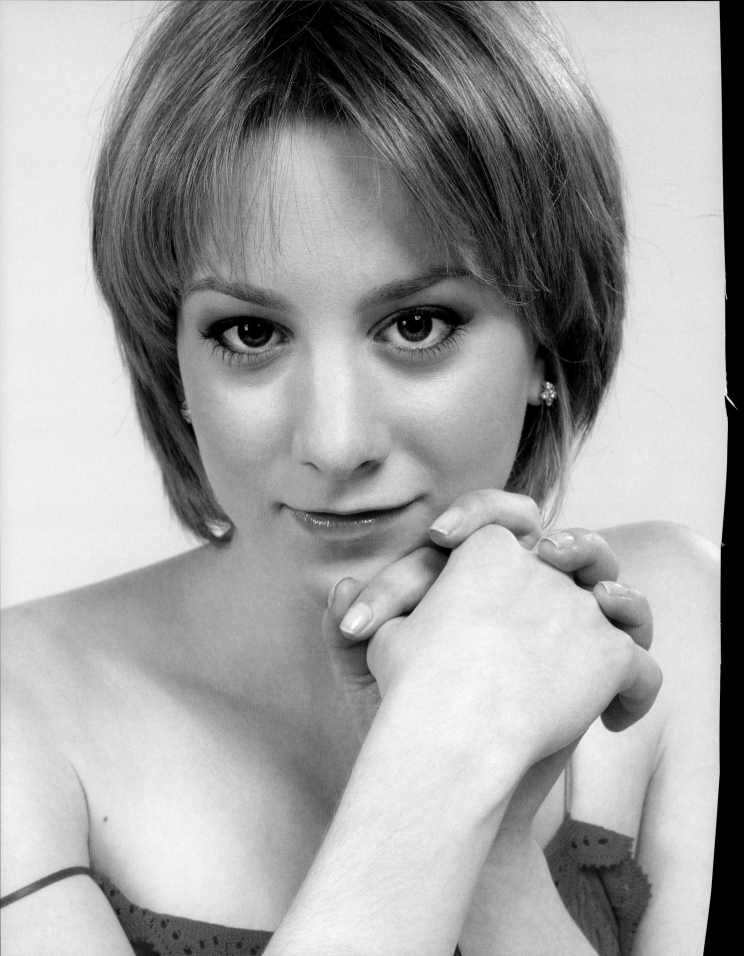

Foreword

by Sarah Hughes,
Olympic Gold Medalist

I was looking forward to February 21, 2002, knowing it would be one of the most important nights of my life. That was the night I hoped to skate for an Olympic gold medal. I had spent endless hours practicing at my rink. My physical and mental conditioning required dedication and caring support from my family, friends, and coach.

After I qualified for the Olympic team in January 2002, my coach and I decided that in order for me to succeed in the Olympics, I still needed some technical advances in my skating program, some changes to my music, new skating dresses—and a new hairstyle that would accent these other changes.

I knew just where to go—Vincent Roppatte at the Elizabeth Arden Salon at Saks Fifth Avenue in New York! Thanks to Vincent, I faced the camera, the media, and skating fans feeling great about my appearance.

Teenagers are always trying for the "perfect hair day." Vincent's book *Cool Hair* provides us with various ways to maximize our self-confidence and to obliterate our bad hair days. What Vincent did for my hair gave me a level of confidence that was the perfect fit for the perfect night. I am sure he has a look for you to complement your individuality. He will give you the know-how to create whatever style your heart desires.

Enjoy reading about all your options and remember—it was Vincent who fashioned the *Sarah Hughes golden hair look*. Have fun with *your* new look and thank you for supporting Vincent's favorite charity—cancer research for children—by buying this book.

Seventeen-year-old Sarah Hughes has been America's darling ever since she astonished the world by skating a joyous, near-perfect program to capture the 2002 Olympic Gold Medal in women's figure skating. The grace she shows on the ice is replicated in her many charitable and business endeavors as she travels the world as a role model for teenagers everywhere. She's our hero, and the pensive, alluring photograph on the preceding page shows another side to this spunky, delightful young athlete.

Cool Hair

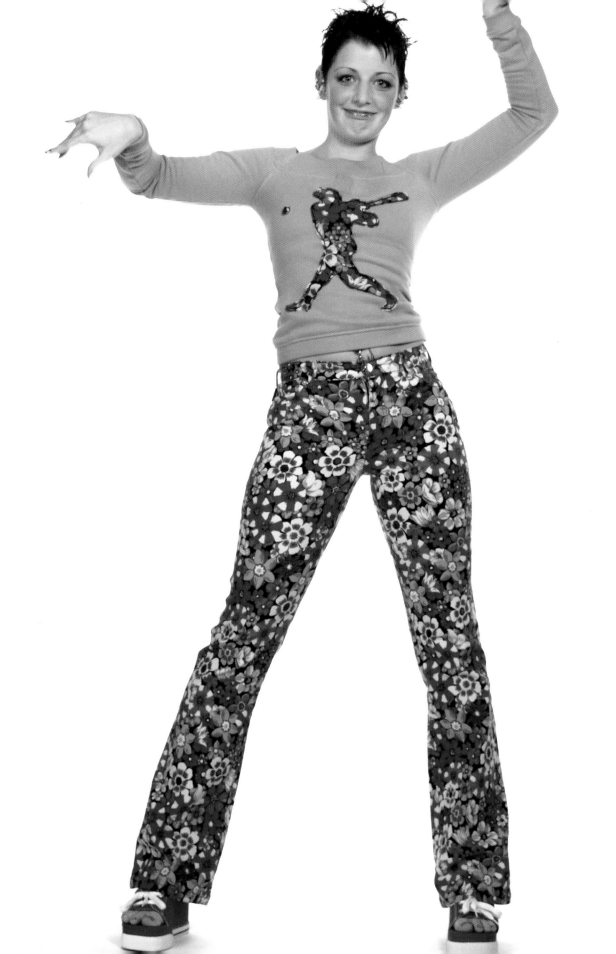

You're the Best | 1

Each and every one of you is a wonder, unique and different from other girls. Although there's a lot more going on inside the private you than anyone dreams, there are still many feelings you share with other teens.

These feelings represent the most important changes in your life, just as you're becoming an irresistible young woman. Can you recognize yourself in the following behaviors?

- You want more privacy than ever before.

- You are easily hurt.

- You want to experiment—look new, try new things, think new thoughts, maybe even *shock* people with your daring.

- Sometimes, you're mean to others—and you regret it.

- Being popular counts—a lot—even if you don't love admitting it.

- Your moods change suddenly.

- Occasionally, you feel anxious about making—and keeping—new friends.

- Your self-esteem flutters—you often don't like yourself and you worry about your appearance.

- You want the right to choose what you wear and how your hair looks.

Even though I'm no expert in psychology, I have spent all my life studying young women and what makes them look wonderful. What I've learned is that it's all about self-esteem and believing in yourself. When you feel confident

Seventeen-year-old Rita Nepogoda is a gentle, free spirit—from her multi-colored toenails to her multiple ear piercings. She follows her dreams and she's the best!

inside, you take on an outside glow and your best qualities show. You don't feel self-conscious about expressing your deepest thoughts. And this I know for sure: The first step toward self-esteem and popularity is feeling comfortable and pretty in your own skin.

Peer pressure can be killing. Although you have definite ideas, it's often easier to be swept along with the crowd and say you like the same bands, clothes, hairstyles, and makeup that everyone else likes, instead of expressing your real opinions. You don't want to be different.

When you don't feel pretty, it's even more difficult to let your true self shine through. If you think you're plain looking, it's harder to relax and be yourself around guys—and even other girls. What you want to say comes out sounding totally lame. Though your achievements, intelligence, and inner qualities best define the person you are, it's easier to believe in yourself if you feel attractive.

People may tell you that thinking about your looks is shallow and unimportant; well, they're wrong, wrong, wrong. Knowing you have the prettiest hair in your class, knowing you're wearing a great outfit don't mean you're shallow. You feel smarter, funnier, and safer if you feel cool. When we know we look good, we attract the best to ourselves and our best selves come out.

Deep inside—you're the best. So what's stopping you from taking control of your outside look and making it the best also? When you do the most with what you have, you'll have the freedom to be yourself inside *and* outside. And I promise you this: One of the best ways to look cool is with wonderful hair that captures the enviable energy and radiance of your youth.

That's why you're holding this book in your hands. If you're not satisfied with the way you look, if you feel out of it, today is the day you change things. Today is the day you start to allow the beauty deep inside you to be set loose.

Reality Check

If you try on the hottest outfit in the world and your hair hangs limp, the effect is also limp, uninteresting. If your hair looks great, so do you—even in your rattiest jeans and T-shirt.

Look at the before and after photos on pages 4–7. Since everyone always talks about bad hair days, we thought we'd see if there is such a thing. We asked some girls who were not particularly happy with the way their hair looked to be photographed. Result? Kind of blah. Then, after a simple makeover, they were photographed again. The results are dynamite—as you can plainly see.

You try it. One day, when your hair is not its best, put on your favorite outfit and look in the mirror. You won't be happy. Then, wash, blow-dry, and style your hair, and put on the same outfit. The difference is amazing—right?

Wonderful clothes are a good start to your day, but it takes some attention to hair—and also to skin and makeup—to make you look sensational.

I believe that you never need to have another bad hair day, even if you're not crazy about the texture, color, or style of your hair.

What Do You Hate About Yourself?

Does your nose seem too big? Do you have too many freckles? Do you think your lips are too thick?

You are what you are. What makes you unique and terrific is *exactly* the shape of your nose and your lips, the individual jut of your chin—all your characteristics that may not fit the bland beauty norm. Cookie-cutter noses are for plastic dolls, not real, young women. The most fabulous young women I know have learned to love and express their differentness by accentuating what makes them stand out from the crowd. Julia Roberts's wide mouth, Reese Witherspoon's sharp chin, and Renée Zellweger's squinty eyes now set the beauty standards, but I bet when they were teenagers, these stars despaired about looking different from everyone else.

"The thing you hate about yourself tends to be the thing that everyone likes about you," said Nicole Kidman to *People* magazine. You can't easily change some things—like height or coloring; your nose, eyes, or ears; the freckles that drive you nuts; and often, your body shape—so it's smart to make the most of those parts and accept them, even if you can't exactly love them.

Even if you can't change anything else, with the tiniest effort you *can* change the most important part of your look—your hair. Hair is the key to everything. Hair softens a square face, reduces a large nose, balances eyes that are too close together or too wide apart. Great hair helps you value even those features you wouldn't have chosen if you were in charge of designing you.

Hair is also a very safe place to experiment. You don't have to diet to extremes or have plastic surgery. Experimenting with hair is as harmless as it is fun. Hate the curl? Straighten it. Hate the straightness? Curl it. Hate the color? Make it blue. Hate the style? Change it. Whatever mistakes you make are not permanent. Nothing is irreversible because that trusty hair will grow back.

Pretty Appeal

If you let me guide you through the pages of this book, I promise you the hair you deserve—no matter what kind of hair you were born with. I promise to teach you the tools, tricks, and skills for your hair so that you can notch up your personal style. I will show you how to have hair appeal—and you will choose the kind of appeal you desire.

Classic Cheerleader

Jenn, fourteen, is in the ninth grade. A varsity cheerleader, she adores competitions.

When she has to concentrate on her jumps full-time, she likes a simple ponytail that moves when she moves.

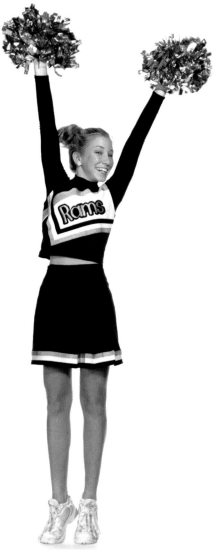

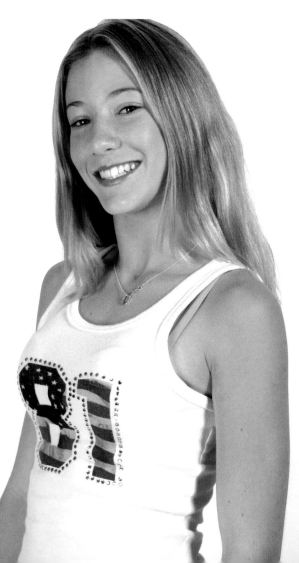

Jenn

Glamour Queen

Lindsay Anderson, eighteen, from Kentucky, was a natural-looking stunner when she appeared in the photography studio.

She's a professional model and knows how to change her look. Here she is a glam queen in an embroidered white jacket and some edgy eye makeup on her beautiful blues.

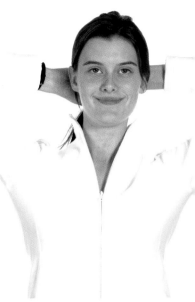

Lindsay

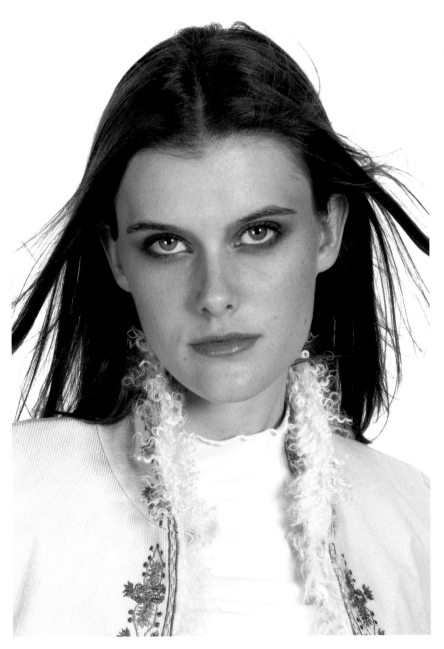

Club Princess

Pretty, seventeen-year-old Lindsay Lohan, star of *Freaky Friday* and *The Parent Trap,* could be your shy best friend in her simple white tank top and jeans.

Clear the dance floor! Now the happening young stunner knows just how to have all the strobe lights focused on her at the club. Her hair is freshly blow-dried, and she's wearing giant hoops, a body-skimming off-the-shoulder jersey, and marvelous attitude!

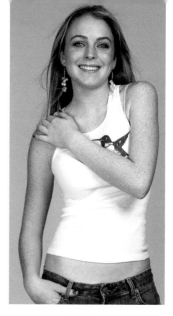

Lindsay

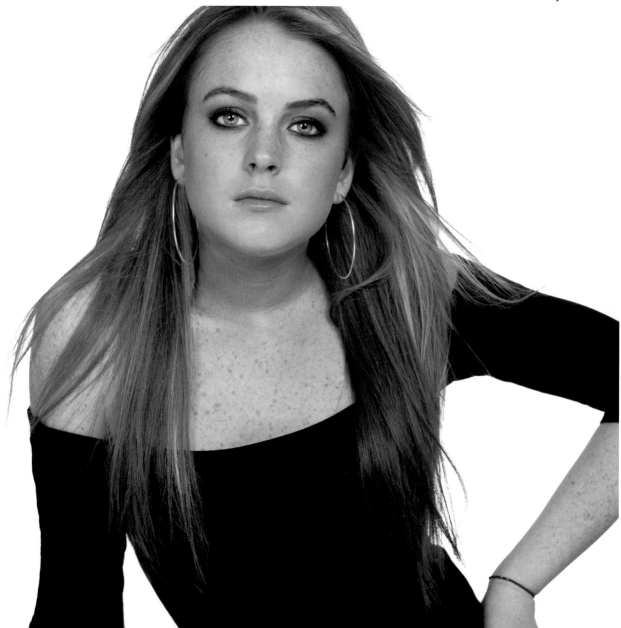

Natural Woman

Keri, sixteen, is a charming, soft-spoken natural beauty with her curly hair caught back in a ponytail.

With blow-dried, straight hair and a smidgen of makeup, she's still a natural beauty—but with enormous style.

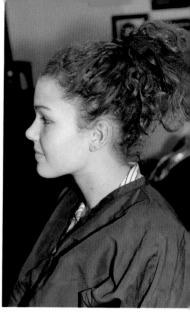

Keri

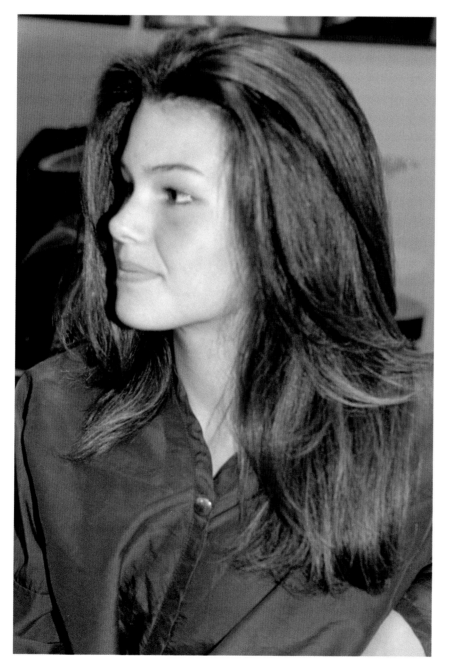

Read My Hair

Sometimes, when you're feeling insecure, you can send silent messages that change the way others perceive you—and those messages can even change the way you feel about yourself. The messages come through your hair.

Have you ever taken a good look at your best friend's face, and, even if she hasn't said a word, you know just what she's thinking? Reading faces is a developed skill. By the time you hit your teens, you're an expert at this kind of nonverbal communication. Have you ever thought about reading hair? Often, the hairstyle a girl chooses on a particular day speaks volumes about what she's thinking or feeling or what she *wants you to believe* she's feeling. You can actually send messages to the world through your hairstyles.

The best thing to do after a crisis—for example, when Mr. Right breaks up with you, you have a fight with your friend, or you bomb out on a chemistry exam—is to change your hairstyle and tell the world you're moving on. The same thing works after a moment of extreme happiness—when you make up with Mr. Right, win a student council election, or make the honor roll. Just as your clothes and your smile send messages of spirit and cool, your new pretty hairstyle also lets the world know you feel great.

The secret is that when you look confident and happy, you get to *feel* that way; it has to do with the way people treat you when they spot your mood. A new hairstyle picks you up and makes you confident. If your hair hangs down lamely and limply, others quickly read that your self-esteem is zero. On the other hand, a shining and bouncy hairstyle will communicate that you have the potential to be funny, fun, and popular (even if you don't always feel that way). When you send out vibes of *pretty* and *interesting* to others, you become appealing. Others want to be with you. People will read your hair, pick up on your self-confidence, and follow you anywhere! When people react to you that way, you yourself become convinced that you're sitting on top of the world. I know this as well as I know hair.

Check the two looks on pages 10 and 11 to see examples of how the world reads your hairstyle choices. Ask your hairstylist for help in creating a style that matches the message you want to send.

Eighteen-year-old Page Stoup's sleek, shining, tawny hair pulled back from her pretty face gives a message of secure self-confidence that seems to say, "I'm ready for anything . . . college, law school, Hollywood starlet, true love! Bring it on!"

The Messages You Might Want Others to Read from Your Hair

I'm just so cute: *"I'm a little shy, but I'd sure like to get to know you. When we're friends, you'll see how cute and appealing I am. . . . Can't you tell by my braids?"*

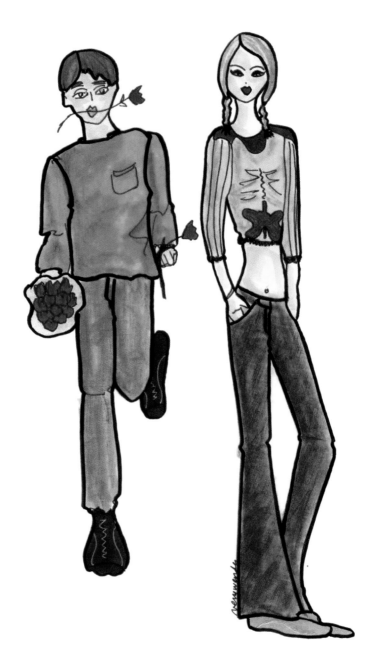

I feel like flirting: *"Hi, new guy. Hi, skateboard hero—I'm your fantasy woman and my cropped hairstyle says I'm all about ease, attitude, and playfulness."*

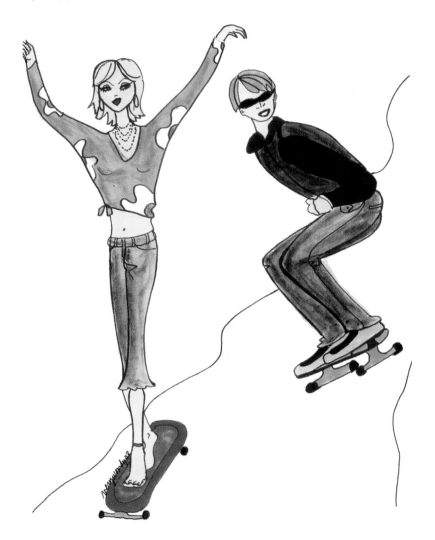

This is the essence of my deeply held belief: Most teens are amazing people who just don't know it yet. The pages that follow are a celebration of teenagers. You have it in your control to feel and look pretty and to develop a winning beauty style, just as you can develop a winning attitude. We're never born with an inner knowledge of how to best blow-dry hair or what to wear to make an impression on an interesting guy. We have to learn the essentials of *pretty,* and, as you read on, I'll show you how to enhance your best natural characteristics as well as make wonderful new choices for the quintessential you. I can do this—trust me! We can do it together.

You're the best.

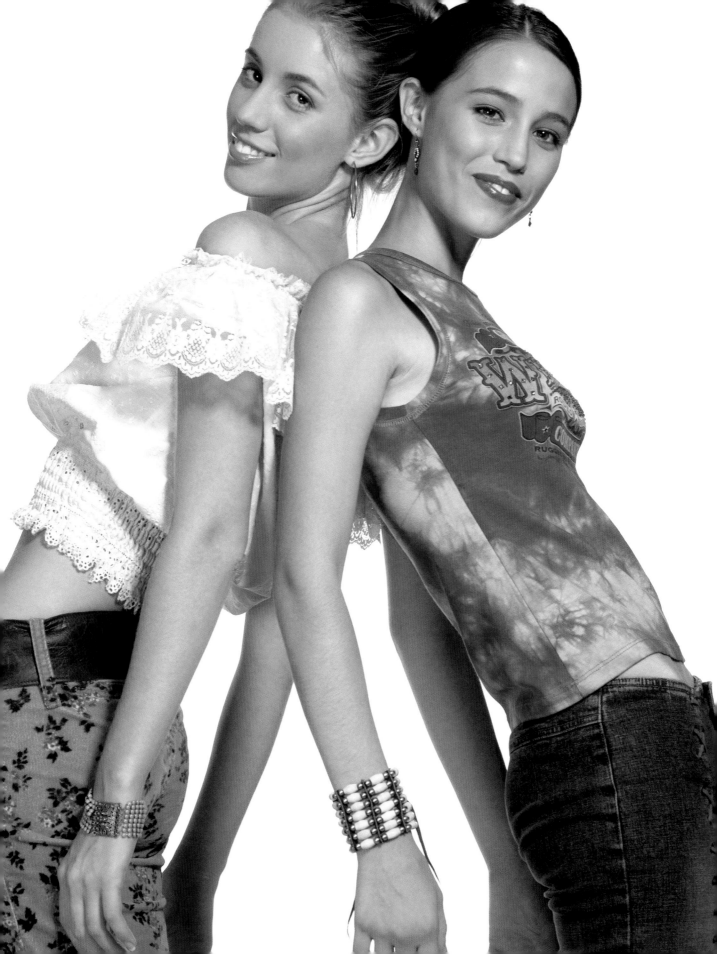

Inside Out | 2

Before you concentrate on how to create a new external look, let's spend a few moments on what's inside. When you see a teenager with fabulous, shining hair, it's a good bet that she's healthy. Nothing you put on your hair, including the most expensive shampoos and conditioners, means anything if you're not healthy. Pretty hair starts on the inside.

Garbage In, Garbage Out

I'm not here to give you boring lectures or draw diagrams of nutritional food pyramids, but savvy teenagers understand that hair doesn't just *grow* from your scalp—it's an integral part of the skin. Since hair is an actual extension of your body, it flourishes when you're healthy and well nourished. Conversely, hair loses its strength and vitality when your body's fed poorly—stuffed with cookies, chips, and Big Macs—or starved because you're perpetually on a punishing diet.

Many models and actresses project an unhealthy and unrealistic view of what a young woman's body should look like. If you're taking your cue about thinness from your favorite superstar, you should know that film and fashion photographs are usually altered by airbrushing or computer manipulation and favorable lighting. If you saw the superstar on the street, you'd probably be shocked by how thin she *isn't*. You might also be surprised to know that the really thin superstar often has serious emotional problems; the stress of having to be skinny and not eat can be unbearable.

Healthy sisters, forever! Eighteen-year-old Alix and thirteen-year-old Victoria.

Food for Thought

The adage "You can never be too thin" is just plain wrong. What is appealing are shapely, healthy young women with an appetite for life, love, and also food—not emaciated, gaunt girls. Stick-figure bodies are just not good-looking, and you need energy to live an exciting life. Food's not the enemy—stringent diets are. They will rob you of your radiance, energy, and health.

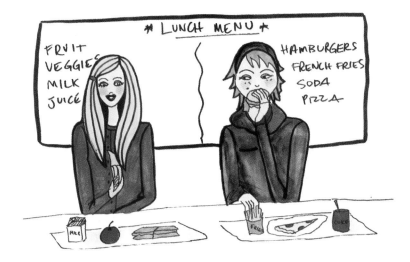

The other extreme's not terrific either. Great hair and skin don't come from stuffing yourself with junk food; an excess of sugar and fat does not add to your glow. Hair becomes thin and brittle, dull and colorless if you don't eat properly. Skin becomes sallow and lackluster or inflamed. You are naturally gorgeous, so eat well to stay that way.

During your teens, your hair has the potential to look better than it ever will at any other time of your life. But during your teens, it's also easier to have limp, greasy-looking hair and more pimple emergencies than at any other time.

It's not *all* about what you eat.

For example, chocolate doesn't give you pimples, no matter what your mother told you. That's one of the great myths about zits. Sweets will never cause your skin to break out or your hair to look limp; your ability to produce oil does it.

Oil City

Teenagers often have special hair and skin problems because natural hormonal changes spur heavy oil production—in some girls more than others.

Although experts agree that teenage stress is partly responsible for bad skin and hair, most believe that these hormone riots are the true culprits. Rising hormone levels cause the oil glands of the skin to enlarge and produce an oily substance called sebum. Sebum, along with various bacteria and flaked-off skin, irritates and clogs skin pores and hair follicles, preventing the oil from draining. For skin, the result is an inflammation, otherwise known as a pimple, and sometimes worse—full-blown acne.

Acne is the result of oil clogging the skin's hair follicles, which is why you get pimples on your face, back, and chest, where hair follicles are found—and not on your palms or the bottoms of your feet, where there are none.

Even if you put mostly good things in your body, oil-producing hormones can still make your face look like a war zone. There are many products that can help. Talk to your physician about your medical options and ask about over-the-counter pore uncloggers that contain benzoyl peroxide or salicylic acid (if you're allergic to aspirin, these products may not be right for you) and topical antibiotics.

Hormones also produce oily hair. This has nothing to do with good or bad health—it has to do with being between thirteen and nineteen years old. This condition won't last forever. In the meantime, I'll give you some advice about caring for oily hair and skin later, in Chapter 9.

Move It!

While we're considering a healthy body's relationship to cool hair, let's not forget exercise. I am a powerful believer in *moving.* It's great for your physical well-being and psyche, but it's also the most effective beauty enhancer I know. In addition to building firm, taut muscles and burning calories, exercise increases blood flow to the skin, and this nourishes facial and scalp cells with oxygen and nutrients. That's very good for your complexion and your hair.

Exercise also removes cellular wastes and encourages your skin to thrive at maximum efficiency. And, even better, exercise makes you feel happy. When we're involved in any pleasurable activity, the brain releases chemical substances called endorphins—the "feel-good" chemicals. Well, those natural highs are produced when you run, swim, ride your bicycle, or indulge in any other form of physical exercise. Exercise beats drinking, smoking, and doing drugs for feel-good benefits.

Want cool hair? For starters, eat well, exercise, educate yourself on how to deal with all that hormonal oil—and it can't hurt to think good thoughts.

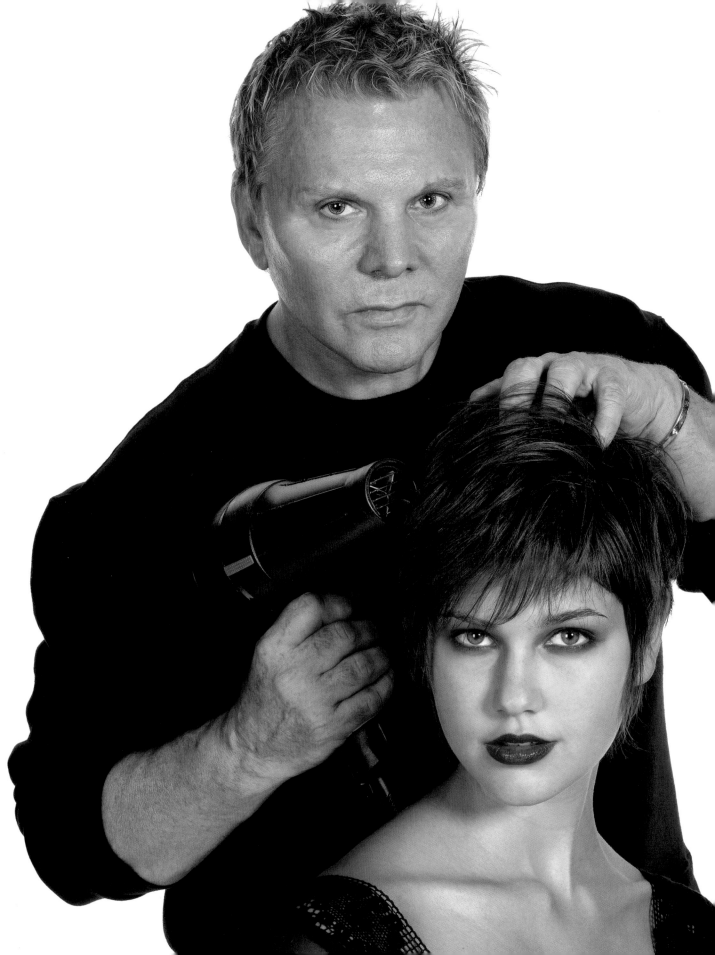

Such Beautiful Hair: | 3
Texture and Care

You can be the girl they're talking about when they whisper, "*She has such beautiful hair*." Before we begin the journey to the essentials of cool hair, take this short quiz to determine what your relationship with hair says about you.

1. How do you usually wear your hair?

   a. with a headband, in a ponytail, or with barrettes—I don't spend more than five minutes a day on it

   b. sleek and straight, curly and wild, or pulled back in a bun—I enjoy messing with different styles, which takes time, but doesn't rule my day

   c. flavor of the day—whatever's new

   d. the color changes very often—depending on my mood

   e. in pretty much the same style every day (since I spend about two hours on hair daily, I'll do anything to avoid messing it up)

2. You are having a really bad hair day. You

   a. don't go to school or to your job

   b. wear a hat or scarf on your hair

   c. mush some gel into your hair and make spikes

   d. slick it back behind your ears or use some interesting clips for damage control

   e. put on a tennis sweatband and concentrate on a great makeup

3. What is the most radical thing you've ever done to your hair?

   a. bleached it

The very beautiful eighteen-year-old Jennifer Coleman and I discuss the way she'd like her hair to look. Result—dynamite!

b. trimmed it

c. got a daring haircut—from long to a boy crop

d. added highlights

e. at least three of the following:
   - shaved your head
   - straightened or permed your tresses
   - let a friend razor-cut it
   - ironed it
   - colored it blue or pink

4. **How do you go about making changes to your hairstyle?**

   a. I never make changes to my hairstyle—well, almost never.

   b. I watch the magazines and films and choose my favorite celebrity style.

   c. I wear the hairstyle that the more popular girls in school choose.

   d. It depends totally on my mood.

   e. My hairdresser decides, or sometimes my mom.

5. **You hate your friend's new haircut like poison. When she asks what you think, you say:**

   a. excellent

   b. fabulous

   c. How do *you* feel about it?

   d. It'll grow back.

6. **You've been invited to a major party. This is what you'll do with your hair:**

   a. the usual—they'll like me the way I am or not at all

   b. blue tips and orange streaks should do it—make all eyes turn to me

   c. ask my hairstylist, "What do you suggest?"

   d. something brand-new but subtle—a new part, maybe

7. **How would Dr. Seuss describe the way your hair looks?**

   a. scraggly, sizzled, French-fried frizzled

   b. bouncy-jouncy, peppy-snappy

   c. to think that I saw it on Dull-Berry Street

   d. droopy, drippy, not so zippy

8. Pull out a hair from the top of your head. When you hold it between your fingers and pull

   a. it breaks in half

   b. it feels dry and brittle and you're sure that it's a split end

   c. it's a beauty!

   d. are you crazy—pull out a hair? Who can spare it?

9. True or false? Put a *T* after every true statement and an *F* after every false one.

   a. Cutting your hair makes it grow in thicker and faster.

   b. The natural texture of your hair won't change throughout your life.

   c. When coloring your hair, your hairdresser (or you) should treat the roots differently from the rest of your hair.

   d. Never, never cut your own split ends—you'll ruin yourself!

   e. Want green hair? Swim in the pool a lot without protecting your hair.

Scoring and Analysis

1. Give yourself 10 points for *a* or *b,* minus 5 points for *c, d,* or *e.*

2. Take 10 points for *c, d,* or *e,* 5 for *b,* and minus 5 for *a.*

3. Take 10 points for *a, b,* or *d,* 5 for *c,* and minus 5 for *e* (you're a little excessive about your hair).

4. Take 10 for *b* or *d,* 5 for *e,* and minus 5 for *c* (you've chosen a style that's popular, not necessarily right for you).

5. Take 10 for *c*—that's the most honest and empathic response. Take 5 for *a* or *b*—they're lies but meant to be kind. Take minus 5 for *d*— that's cruel.

6. Take 10 for *d,* 5 for *c,* 2 for *b,* and 0 for *a* (you sound a little unadventuresome—maybe insecure? You're not dampening your individuality appeal by looking as pretty as you can).

7. Take 10 for *b,* 5 for *c,* and minus 5 for *a* or *d.*

8. Take 10 for *c,* 5 for *a* or *b* (you need some work), and minus 5 for *d* (this is a danger signal—you need *serious* work).

9. a. Take 10 for an *F* response. It may look thicker when shorter and may seem to grow in faster—but it isn't and it doesn't.

b. Take 10 for an *F* response. Lots of factors may change your hair's texture permanently or temporarily, like medication, age, or pregnancy.

c. Take 10 for a *T* response. The new hair coming in absorbs color much faster than already treated hair.

d. Take 10 for an *F* response. Sure, you can cut a bit off—with a good scissors.

e. Take 10 for a *T* response. The Chlorine is murder on hair, often turning it green. Use a thick coat of conditioner over your hair every time you swim in a pool.

Did you score from 90 to 110? Call up the shampoo-commercial people this minute—you're the new star! Your hair is healthy and pretty, and you have a knowledgeable attitude about its care. Sure, you love great-looking hair and you pay attention and time to the way it looks and feels—it is, after all, the number one beauty asset of any teen—but you're not obsessed with it. You are cautious about sun and chemical damage so you don't overdo either. Best of all, you understand the value of maintenance.

Did you score from 50 to 85? I'll bet your hair looks good much of the time, but you need to rethink the amount of time you spend (or don't spend) on it— something's a tad off. And, frankly, you don't seem to be all that savvy about hair health and how to treat problems. I like that you're not frantic about always looking perfect. No one ever does and it's pointless to disappear on bad hair days. After you read further, you'll score higher.

Did you score under 50? Not a terrific score. Hair's not your crowning glory yet. Still, if you're desperate about the way your hair looks, you can always visit a great hairstylist if only to get a great cut—and that will solve many problems. Also, if you've chemically overtreated your hair, it will grow back healthy and you can start fresh and become more sophisticated about its care and feeding. Read on.

My Private Style Formula

Einstein had his formula of relativity: $E = MC^2$. I have my own formula: $S = TC^3$. Translated, that means: **style equals texture times care, cut, and color.**

Having great hair is very different from being trendy or fashionable; having a great hair style means that you carry your own style with you even though fashion and trends change every five minutes. Having great style makes you the focus of admiration. It is more important than having great cheekbones. Great style commands attention. It is a statement about yourself. Fashion is what manufacturers and beauty directors decide will be popular each year. Style is what *you* decide is marvelous for you. If your style is unique and personal, it will shine through your life.

It takes energy, self-knowledge, and an interest in the world to develop true style, but when you get it down, people will recognize it.

Part You / Part Invention

Style involves inventing a great look by working with what you have and making the most of it, and also taking some calculated risks.

Britney Spears found her signature hairstyle—that long, swingy look that's perfect for her naturally straight hair. She might be trendier with a chopped, blunt cut, but that simply isn't her style—and she wouldn't look as sensual. Of course, she's added great, delicate layering to her hair as well as some strategically placed highlights, and her partly natural/partly invented look is fabulous.

Halle Berry instinctively knew that her personal best is a short, boy crop. It's hard to think of her with any other look. Boy crop is her style—she owns it.

You may try to copy the sleek, straight style of Gwyneth Paltrow's or Jennifer Aniston's hair, but if you were born with Sarah Jessica Parker's ringlets or Beyoncé Knowles's huge, curly mane—even if you reinvent yourself by having your hair straightened—long, straight hair is never going to work very well for you. You can, however, take moderate risks with color and texture changes that give you a fresh look as long as you keep the right balance.

Here's where my formula comes in (**style equals texture times care, cut, and color**). To find the best *style* for you, go through the formula, one step at a time.

Style=
    Texture ×
        Care
            Cut
                Color

First, let's pinpoint *texture* to identify what kind of hair you have naturally. You need to know that so you can get the proper *care, cut,* and *color* for it.

Texture

Determining Your Hair Texture

The feel of your hair is what's commonly known as its texture. The consistency and shape of each single hair on your head, together with the amount of hair on your head, constitute its texture. Once you know what texture hair you have, you can start a plan of action to care for your hair. How often you shampoo or condition your hair depends on its texture.

Coarse, Fine, or Medium Hair

Coarse hair: If your hair is coarse, each single hair will feel substantial and thick—not wispy or delicate. If you put coarse hair in a ponytail, it will feel wonderfully bouncy and wiry, not silky and limp. It's hard to run a brush through coarse hair, particularly if it's curly. Just to give you a reference, Asian hair is usualy coarse and straight.

Fine hair: If your hair is fine, it feels like baby's hair—silky and flyaway. Fine hair is exquisite to touch but sometimes difficult to style because it doesn't have much natural body and almost never stands away from your face. Your ponytail will feel supersoft but sometimes be limp. When you lift your head from the pillow in the morning, your fine hair will probably be clinging to your face.

Medium hair: If your hair is medium, most of your styling and care worries are over. Medium hair is the easiest to work with. Still, your hair texture can be different depending on the weather and your own body temperature and condition. A humid day or an illness can cause your medium-textured hair to hang a little droopingly. A cool day makes your hair feel more substantial and wiry. You know your hair is medium textured if it takes a blow-dry and a set very well. The hair dries with bounce and volume, and a set holds and lasts, at least throughout the day.

Oily or Dry Hair

Whether your hair is oily or dry is another key component of texture.

Oily hair: Your hair is oily if it looks flat and greasy when you don't wash it daily. Often, it feels slippery and slick to the touch. If you blow-dry it when it's not perfectly clean, your hair will be difficult to style and your set will not hold.

But oily hair, when cared for properly, can have the look of really gorgeous, healthy, lustrous hair. Most teens have oily hair because of their increased hormone production, but as they get older, miraculously, much of that oil seems to disappear.

Dry hair: Your hair is dry if it feels brittle, looks fuzzy and strawlike, and breaks easily when you don't condition it. It's often flyaway messy and has a tendency to look dull. Girls with dry hair usually have split ends—hairs that are frayed at the ends. These splits, if not trimmed off, unravel—the split travels up the hair shaft, producing a sloppy and wispy appearance. The plus side of dry hair is that, when properly conditioned, it takes a set and styling beautifully.

Dry hair and dry scalp are often associated with dandruff—those white flakes that flutter down from the hair in an embarrassing snowfall. Dandruff doesn't come from dry hair or scalp at all but usually from an increased production of skin cells—a condition formally known as seborrheic dermatitis. Stress and seasonal changes can induce the condition. If dandruff is a problem, use an over-the-counter dandruff shampoo or ask your dermatologist to prescribe a cream that's just right for your hair type. *Tip:* Beware of product buildup. An overdose of styling products may also be the culprit when it comes to those little white flakes.

Thin, Full, or Average Hair

The amount of hair on your head—whether it's a lot, a little, or average—is also a component of texture and how your hair feels. Most girls average about 100,000 hairs on their heads, and it's natural to lose about 100 hairs daily as you go about brushing, washing, and hot-air drying your hair.

Thin hair: Some healthy girls just naturally have fewer hairs. You'll know you're one of those girls if your hair feels slightly unsubstantial and scanty, but it covers your head evenly. A good hairdresser can give you a cut to make your hair look and feel fuller. Sometimes, you can give thin hair to yourself. If you've relentlessly been pulling your hair into a tight ponytail or using a hot comb, very harsh chemicals, very tight curlers, or a very hot blow-dryer too close to your head, you may notice little bald spots scattered over your head. This kind of thinning hair is not natural, and it can be fixed if you stop inflicting damage before scar tissue forms.

Finally, *and this is very rare,* sometimes very young women can have thinning hair due to genetics, stress, or illness. This condition is known as alopecia and can often be treated by a physician.

Full hair: Sometimes, girls actually have more than 100,000 hairs on their heads, usually of an exceptionally coarse, curly character. You'll know you have a very full head of hair if it's difficult to gather in a clip and it takes forever to blow-dry. When styled properly, full hair looks simply marvelous; but, again, very full hair must be carefully shaped so that it doesn't look wild and unkempt.

Medium or average hair: Your hair amount is medium, or average, if it is supple and substantial but easy to handle. It doesn't feel particularly thin or thick. Lucky girl.

Texture Transformations

You say you hate your coarse, curly hair like poison—and the limited number of styles that come along with it? You say your straight, fine hair is a bother, you want more body, and are tired of losing the battle?

If you've tried all the looks appropriate to your natural hair texture and are unhappy, you can change your look by altering the texture of your hair. There have been so many advances and developments in hair care, you don't have to live with the hair texture you hate.

Before You Take the Plunge

Don't try this at home. You *must* go to a professional for a texture change—a perm or straightening—because the chemicals involved are strong and potentially dangerous.

Get a new haircut *after* your perm or straightening: The new texture will call for a different kind of cut and style. And, remember, nothing lasts forever. As your hair grows, the roots will have their natural texture. Unless you keep getting those chemical treatments, you may have to rethink that cut. Curly roots of straightened hair look strange when they grow back, so you have to be really vigilant about redoing the roots.

Don't do two things at once; go for the texture change first. Wait to get your hair colored (if you color it) for at least forty-eight hours after the texture change. If you color your hair first, the texture process may change the color.

If your scalp is sensitive or if you have broken skin in any area on the scalp, postpone having the texture change to avoid skin irritation.

You must use regular, deep conditioning on straightened or permed hair to keep it soft and to prevent tangles. Good conditioners keep static electricity to a minimum—the biggest cause of flyaway hair—and give hair a wonderful shine.

Here's a thought: If you have a hairstylist who's willing to take the time to experiment with different looks for you, *before* you have a serious texture change, go for it. Although it won't last, sometimes just a set with fatter rollers and a good blow-dry will show you, for example, how your curly hair could look with a permanent texture change.

Types of Texture Changes

Perming

A permanent curls the hair by using chemicals, along with rollerlike rods, to change your straight texture and create a curly or wavy one. A perm lasts about three to four months. Your own stylist may use a different process or a combination of processes, but here are a number of traditional curling options:

Regular perm: The entire head of hair gets curled. It can be more curly or less curly, depending on the rod size and number of rods used. Fat rods give a loose curl; thin ones give a tight curl.

Root perm: Curling rods are placed only at the roots of the hair to give volume, body, or "lift."

Spot perm: Curl is added by placing rods only in places where you want more fullness.

Body wave: Large, fat rods are used to give a soft curl.

Straightening

If your hair is naturally very curly, frizzy, or kinky and you don't like it or just want to experiment with a new look, you can have your hair chemically straightened, or "relaxed." Remember that the chemicals used can severely damage your hair. Go to a professional—I can't recommend that strongly enough unless bald is the look for you. Here are some options:

Straightening: Powerful chemicals are used to make your hair really straight. Hair straightening usually lasts from four to six months, but when the roots first become noticeable—usually in two to three months—your stylist can apply relaxer to the new growth only. The previously straightened hair must be protected with a heavy conditioner during this touch-up.

Relaxing: Less powerful chemicals reduce your curls to straightness. You might consider relaxing only the underneath layer of your hair. The curls on top will not stick out as much if the hair underneath is straight.

Bio-ionic relaxing: A trendy, Asian-invented chemical process that makes the hair bone-straight and very easy to blow-dry and style. I will only use it on virgin hair, which has never seen chemicals or color. The downside is that this process is very expensive and more time-consuming than any other hair relaxer. Note: The strong chemicals must never touch the scalp during application, to avoid burns.

Texturing: Relaxer chemicals are combed through the hair and left on for only a short while to loosen tight curls.

Soft curling: A combination of relaxer chemicals and perm rods are used to reshape and soften curly hair.

Any of these processes can take from two to four hours, including a shampoo and blow-dry, so if you're going for a texture change, clear your schedule.

Care

Once you know your hair's texture—either its natural texture or the texture you've chosen by perming, straightening, or relaxing—you must determine the proper cleansing and conditioning care for your hair.

I've noted some of my favorite hair-care products in the following discussion of hair texture, and let's be candid: Supplies can be costly. You should know that the hairstylist's best friend is the beauty supply house, where shampoos, conditioners, sprays, styling products, hair dryers—you name it—are available at big discounts. You can find these listed under Beauty Supplies in the Yellow Pages. Try to save up your needs and make a reasonably substantial purchase when you go. The Manhattan beauty supply house I use is Ray's Beauty Supply Company. Tell them Vincent sent you.

A few words about shampoos: They are not equal. Some have more cleansing and foaming agents (surfactants); some have built-in conditioners; some have thickeners, fragrance, and even chemicals that are supposed to prevent residue buildup. All contain at least 50 percent water. Your goal should be to find a shampoo that won't strip your hair of its good natural oils along with the dirt and won't be heavy with the additives that can make the hair soft but also limp. Experimenting is the only way to find the best product for you.

And one caution about both shampoos and conditioners: Don't use too much—which generally means using less than the instructions on the bottle advise. You can even dilute a bottle of conditioner with water, creating double the amount. Too much and too strong a conditioner generally make for limp hair.

Let's Begin

Coarse Hair

If you have coarse hair, shampoo it as often as necessary—even twice a day if you're very athletic and perspire a lot. Use a moisturizing, fortifying shampoo which contains ingredients that replenish the hair's moisture; I like *Phytorhum Rum and Egg*. Condition your hair after every shampoo. Try products that contain silicone, an ingredient that smooths and seals the hair cuticle, the outermost layer of the hair, keeping in the moisture that makes your hair soft and keeping out humidity that makes hair frizzy. Very coarse hair often does well with leave-in conditioners. Try *619 Extra Strength Conditioner* by Belair Beauty to see if it works for you. Lanolin drops—a fatty substance obtained from wool and applied after a shampoo—are good for hair that's particularly frizzy. Buy the drops in beauty supply shops. For excellent styling control, a protein pack or hot oil treatment (warm olive oil works well) can be applied to coarse, dry, unwashed hair for twenty minutes once a week; then rinse hair and condition.

Special treatments: I like a slicker that can tame coarse hair into a smooth, shining updo like Frédéric Fekkai's *Pomade Cristal*. Coarse hair holds well with a hair spray that's not gluey or sticky, like Mario Tricoci's fine mist *Sculpting Spray,* which can be used on wet or dry hair. Elizabeth Arden and other fine salons, in addition to beauty supply stores, carry Tricoci products.

Fine Hair

If you have fine hair, use a protein shampoo like Privé's *Laurent D. Extreme Volume* (with volume-building elements like panthenol and protein) every other day. Once a week, you can also try an amplifying (sometimes called volumizing) shampoo (Physique puts out a good one) that contains water-attracting ingredients that swell the hair shaft and pump up the hair. Amplifying shampoos can leave a residue that weighs down fine hair, so alternate them with a regular shampoo.

Cream rinses are out for you because they soften and weigh down the hair, leaving fine hair limp. Try an herb-based conditioner twice weekly.

Special treatments: Hair color adds volume, so if you're thinking of some highlights anyway, they will have that added benefit for your fine hair. If you need volume in a hurry, pour a bit of baby powder in your hands and sprinkle it on the roots of your hair: Then, use a paddle brush to back comb at the roots. Finish by smoothing over till the powder is invisible.

Medium Hair

Shampoo medium hair as often as you like and experiment with any shampoo that catches your eye. You should also condition after every shampoo — your flexible hair texture allows you to try many products until you find one you love. Your medium hair may need styling products on humid days. Try Mario Tricoci's *3P-1 Styling Cream,* a three-in-one product for conditioning, smoothing, and shine. The *Paste Hair Holder,* which looks and feels like the white stuff you used in nursery school, is terrific for creating twisted and chunky styles. Note that a tiny dollop of any styling product goes a long way.

Special treatments: For occasional perfect cleanliness, try a clarifying shampoo that has acidic ingredients to strip away excess oils and built-up residues left by other styling products. Use small amounts of clarifying shampoo as it has no conditioning properties and can be harsh. A fifteen-minute protein pack every month gives your medium hair magnificent body and shine. I like the *Phytocitrus Hydrating* product.

Oily Hair

Use an alcohol-free, sebum-cleansing shampoo once or twice a week. *Phytocédrat* is a good product. Try to avoid conditioners, but if you must, use a very light one like *Phytobaume Light Untangling Balm* just at the ends of the hair and only once a week.

Special treatments: For instant oil relief, dip your fingertips in colorless, organic body powder (buy it at the health food store) or even baking soda, massage it into the roots of your hair, then brush to remove. The powder absorbs the oil.

For oily, greasy-looking bangs, spot-treat by sprinkling a bit of dry shampoo (or body powder) on the roots, then brushing it out.

Dry Hair

Don't shampoo your hair more than three to four times a week unless your hair's very dirty. I like a product called *Phytojoba Intense Hydrating Shampoo* for dry hair. If you have dandruff, it probably is not caused by dry scalp (see page 23). If you use a dandruff shampoo, avoid those containing sulfur, which can burn your scalp and hair, unless it's prescribed by a dermatologist. Use a good moisturizing after shampoo treatment like *Phytosésame Detangling Intense Hydrating Cream*. Between hair washes, you can deep-condition once weekly with a protein conditioner. Leave it on for twenty minutes under a damp, warm towel, then rinse.

Special treatments: Make your own protein conditioner by mixing two egg yolks with one tablespoon of sesame oil. Work this into your hair, then cover for twenty minutes with a damp, hot towel. Wash hair thoroughly afterward. For extra shine, add four drops of olive oil to your regular conditioner. Leave it in for about twenty minutes, then rinse out.

Thin Hair

If your hair is thin, try a protein, volume-maximizing shampoo like *Phytovolume* four or five times weekly. Condition sparingly, no more than twice weekly, and then use a protein conditioner with body-building ingredients like balsam or resin. Use a product, like Wella *Liquid Hair Style Builder Phytovolume Actif,* to increase volume, eliminate frizz, and leave hair very glossy.

Special treatments: When styling with a warm blow-dryer, hair mousse mushed evenly through wet roots works very well to give thin, limp hair a thicker appearance. I also like very much the Mario Tricoci *Thickener and Texturizing Cream,* which adds body and promotes natural-looking curls.

Full or Thick Hair

Use a daily shampoo (experiment to find the one that works well) and an all-purpose after shampoo treatment like *Phytobaume*. I like a mild, nondetergent product like *Phytoneutre* shampoo (it won't lather up that much because there's no soap in it).

Special treatments: Use a synthetic-bristle brush if your hair's very thick and tends to tangle. It's stronger than natural bristle and gets rid of knots more easily. Thick hair tends to get out of hand. Two great styling products are Aveda's *Custom Control* and Sebastian's *Pomade*: they give smooth texture and shining control. Use only a pea-size dollop of either and soften the thick consistency by rubbing it between your hands before smoothing down your hair. On a humid day, these products are great for emergency slick backs and funky twists. If you wish to give a flat-ironed effect to the ends of your hair, try a product like Sebastian's *Shaper Hand Press Flattening Fluid*.

Curly Hair

Use very mild shampoos like Biolage products or Bed Head's *Control Freak Shampoo* (*"Stomps the curl and fights the frizzies"*). If you like, you can shampoo daily, but many girls with very curly hair say they shampoo only about twice a week. If you feel strange about not washing your hair daily, you can thoroughly wet it down with water every day to revive your curls. A moisturizing conditioner like Pantene products or Bed Head's *Moisture Maniac Conditioner* should follow each shampoo or wetting.

Special treatments: Revlon puts out a wonderfully inexpensive all-in-one shampoo and conditioner called *Cream of Nature* that's perfect for curly, dry hair. Believe it or not, some of my curliest-haired clients, whose hair is not particularly oily, rarely use shampoo; they "wash" their hair by rubbing their scalps with a teaspoon of a conditioner laden with emollients and humectants (which attract water from the air into the scalp). The tighter the curl in your hair, the more conditioner you need. Two applications, three or four times a week, and your hair is squeaky clean. For very oily, curly hair, use the gentlest, alcohol-free shampoo you can find and, if you must, a clarifying oil-stripping shampoo (see page 38 for a natural clarifying shampoo recipe) no more than once a week. A product called *Phytodéfrisant Hair Straightening Balm* enables you to blow-dry even very curly hair to smooth perfection. Use a product like Bed Head's *Power Trip Hair Gel* to mold and shape curly hair into submission after each shampoo or wetting. I love a botanical nonaerosol holding spray called *Phytolaque* for curly heads. Finally, when drying your hair, use the cool air option of your hair dryer.

Straight Hair

A pure castile soap shampoo works very well; also use a detangler instead of a conditioner. Mario Tricoci's *Hold and Shine Spray* can be used as a softener/detangler on wet hair. For straight hair, I like a botanical product like *Phytolaque,* which gives a soft hold without the stickiness of most hair sprays.

Special treatments: A cold-water final rinse gives great shine. Phyto's *Sculpting Gel* gives great holding power and allows you to shape, spike, or slick back your straight hair. If you want a wet look, just use a little more gel.

Kinky or Frizzy Hair

Use a moisturizing, protein-rich shampoo (try Paul Mitchell *Instant Moisture Daily Shampoo* or any product containing shea butter) at least twice

Your frizzy hair can look just wonderful. Check out Carlotta opposite.

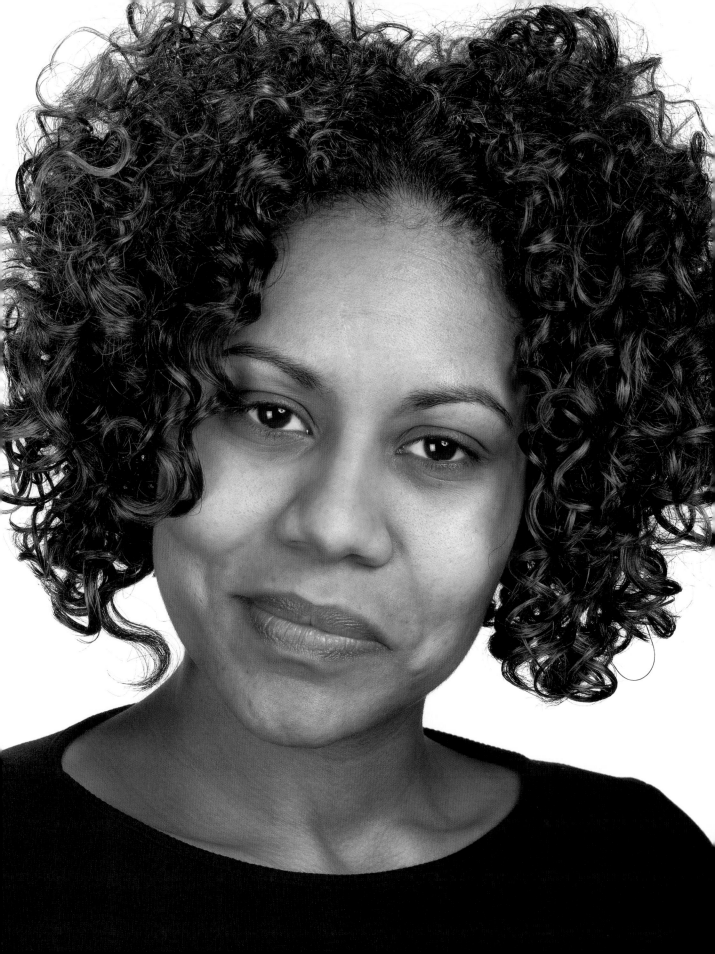

weekly. Use Phytologie *Detangling Balm,* Nexxus *Ensure Acidifying Conditioner and Detangler,* or John Frieda *Frizz-Ease Wind-Down Relaxing Crème* after every shampoo.

Special treatments: Apply several drops of antifrizz, shine serum (like *Frizz-Ease*) to a fat, fluffy makeup brush and brush over hair for frizz control and great shine. Wella *Lifetax Personal Trainer* is another fierce frizz controller. Many clients love to massage the contents of two vitamin E oil capsules into their scalp weekly; they comb it through, sit under a hot, damp towel for fifteen minutes, then rinse very well.

Chemically Treated Hair
(Dyed, Bleached, Straightened, or Permed)

I suggest using a mildly acidic shampoo with built-in protein conditioners as often as needed. *Phytocitrus Vital Radiance* works well, and so does Mario Tricoci's *Shampoo for Dry and Chemically Treated Hair*. You might use a moisturizing conditioner like *Phytocitrus Vital Radiance Mask* (even if your shampoo has built-in protein conditioners) after every shampoo and weekly warm oil treatments.

Special treatments: Color lasts longer if you rinse your hair in cool water. Mario Tricoci's *Uni-Pak Deep Conditioner* contains protein and botanical extracts that repair hair damaged from too much color and blow-drying. A wonderful light holding spray for chemically processed hair is *Phytolaque Soie*. Most important of all, use a shampoo specially formulated for colored, permed, or processed hair: It won't strip the color, as do many other shampoos.

The Cleansing Touch

The process of shampooing is just as important as the product you use. Your hair must be shampooed properly for the best results. Remember—shampoo is not whipped cream. The primary function of shampoo is to clean, so don't confuse cleaning with the amount of lather a shampoo produces. More lather means more detergent, which can dry and dull hair. The real secret to really clean hair is to rinse out all the shampoo.

For easier comb throughs, try combing your hair while the shampoo is still in—*then,* rinse.

Here is the best hair wash in town:

1. First, brush your hair to loosen dirt and tangles and remove shed hairs.

2. Wet your hair with warm water. Squirt the shampoo into your hands—not directly in your hair. Use an amount the size of a quarter for short hair, slightly more for longer hair. Rub your hands together.

3. With your fingers, massage shampoo in small circles into the roots of the hair and your scalp—the most important part of the shampoo. Then lather up the rest of the hair. You need only one shampoo application—no matter what the bottle says.

4. Rinse thoroughly. Rinse again.

5. Put a dollop of conditioner about the size of a nickel in your palms (more for long hair) and rub your hands together. Massage conditioner into the roots and comb through your hair with your fingers.

6. Rinse once with warm water.

7. Now—and this is so important—rinse with water as cold as you can stand for the shiniest hair in town.

8. Comb hair with a wide-toothed comb, towel it dry—and you're ready to blow-dry and style.

The Finishing Touch: Blow-Drying

There is no hair technique more important than blow-drying. Pay close attention to the way the professional stylist does it and ask for advice on how to do it yourself at home. Even if you can't go to a professional, these next sections may be the most useful styling advice in the book.

There are many ways to blow-dry hair. If you've had a very good haircut, and your hair is short, it may be enough just to bend your head forward and down, and move the airflow from the blow-dryer through the hair until it's reasonably dry. Use a flat brush and brush in different directions, even against the part. Then, straighten up. If your hair's been cut well, the layers will lock into place but still look a little tousled, which is sexy and wonderful. Put a little mousse or styling gel on your fingers and gently place your hair in the style you love.

For longer hair and more control over your styling, many young women prefer using a round vent brush or a round bristle brush to style. Here's how to do it:

1. Rub no more than a teaspoonful of mousse or setting lotion between your hands and work it through your wet hair. This will create volume in

the finished style. Remember—less is more. If you use too much product, your hair will be stiff as a board.

2. Use a professional grade blow-dryer (at least 1,600 to 1,875 watts) set to medium heat for quick drying without burning. Wave the dryer over your hair until the hair is about half dry.

3. It's important to blow-dry your hair in sections to get maximum volume and a stable foundation that will allow the style to last. With a long hair clip, take a one-inch section of hair from the top of your head and fasten it out of the way. Then, also clip small sections of hair from the sides of your head, to the top of your head. Leave the hair at the temples and the back of the head loose.

4. At the back of your head at your neck, wind a section of hair over a round brush, pulling the hair up and away from the scalp. Aim the hot air from the dryer at the roots, particularly if you want volume, and pay as much attention to them as to the hair that's wound around the brush.

5. When you think the brush-load of hair is dry, turn the dryer away but don't remove the brush for a few seconds until the hair cools. It takes more time to do it this way, but you get an infinitely better set. If your hair's long enough, you can leave a brush with hair that's tightly wound around it in place, while you work on another section with another brush. I call that *hair acupuncture*—and it works beautifully to set the curl.

6. Continue drying each section of hair. After each section is dried, don't brush out the curls just yet. Wait until your whole head is finished.

7. Last, blow-dry the top section of your hair—the one you first clipped up.

8. Finally, when all your hair is cool, brush and style it as you like. If you need more height on the top or sides, tease the hair a bit. Teasing (or back-combing) is accomplished by combing small hair sections with gentle strokes up toward the roots, then smoothing out the top, creating additional volume or height.

9. If your hair is very curly, you may want to use a diffuser attachment on your blow-dryer. The blower dries the hair as the diffuser gives volume and keeps the curls intact and unfrizzy.

10. My personal trick: Use a light spray to keep your style in place. If you prefer a very natural look, spray your fingers—not your hair—then run your hands over the hair. This works on those cowlicks. Then, comb

your fingers through your hair, styling as you go. Spray, applied in this manner, always makes your hair look and feel more natural.

The Tool Chest

Every girl needs her basic hair tools. It's a good idea to stake out some territory for the tools to live in—perhaps a large hat box or a real tool chest. Keep your combs and brushes clean. Use a comb to remove hair from the brushes,

Model Tips on Blow-drying—and Making It Last

You've gone to all that trouble blow-drying your hair, so you want it to last longer than three minutes. My model clients use all these techniques:

- Blow-dry starting at the root of the hair—not the end or middle. The hair roots are the foundation for the style—and, just like a house, when the foundation is sturdy, the house is solid and will last.

- Smooth laminate drops like *Frizz-Ease Hair Serum* over the hair before you dry it, to seal the cuticle (the outer layer) and make it impervious to humidity. The blow-dried hair will take longer to get flyaway messy.

- Make the blow-dry style last by switching your part. The area along the part gets oily and frizzy first because it's exposed to the air. If you part your hair on one side while you blow-dry it, part it on the other side or in the middle for the next couple of days. Your blow-dried do will last longer.

- The better the body, the longer the last. Rub a dab of gel or mousse between your hands and work through your wet hair. Wind your hair over a round brush, then blow-dry. Then, section off and set the hair for only about ten minutes on fat Velcro rollers. When you comb out to style, you'll have a fuller, stronger, longer-lasting style.

- Back comb your blow-dried hair at the roots to make your style last all night if you're going to a hot, sweaty club or party.

- Apply styling products to the roots, not the ends, of the hair to stop your hair from getting flat.

- Keep your hands out of your hair and your hair out of your face. Oils can be transferred from face and hands to hair, causing havoc to freshly blow-dried hair. Keep your skin very clean and even use a headband at home to keep your bangs from absorbing skin oil.

then soak the brushes and combs for ten minutes in a mixture of hot water and shampoo. Rinse in warm running water. Keep your curlers, clips, and rollers well organized in their own separate containers. Here are my choices:

Brushes

I like the Denman curling brushes, which come in all sizes. They smooth and straighten curly hair or create curls in straight hair. Each size brush comes with ten rows of bristles and a natural wooden handle. The company also offers a synthetic-bristle brush for very coarse hair.

The curlier your hair, the bigger the brush you should use. I also like the metal-bodied round brushes put out now by every company in the world, but Paul Mitchell does it best with the *Scalpmaster*. The holes in the metal base act like air vents, and the metal holds the heat amazingly well when you style to curl or straighten. Mason Pearson hairbrushes are classics. I always carry a pocket-sized one.

For removing tangles, try the Paul Mitchell *Superbrush 427*.

For styling very long hair, you must have a large—at least three-inch—boar-bristle brush.

Use a wide, flat, paddle brush to straighten, gloss, and even polish the hair. Paddle brushes are very good for drying long hair that's straight or wavy, but the flat base can't create the pull needed to straighten curly hair. The best ones have the bristles set in a rubber cushion.

Combs

How would I live without the vintage, fine-toothed tail comb that has been around forever? It's used for back-combing hair. For me, the tail is the only way to create a perfect part.

The lift pick is also terrific—it's a comb with a double pronged handle. Insert the prongs into the hair where you need volume or height, lift, then spray the hair.

Straightening Tools

I love the flat iron—it's a marvelous tool. Just place small, combed-through sections of dry hair between the two flat heated paddles and glide the iron from the roots to the ends (pull downward rather than out). Watch straightening magic happen to curly hair.

Tape a double tissue under the flat iron on your scalp, so you don't burn yourself, even a little.

Don't iron hair more than twice weekly or you'll fry it.

Curlers

- Velcro rollers attach to the hair without clips or pins. They now come in electric models.

- Heated rollers (the smaller rollers give the tightest curls, the fatter ones give the looser, more natural curls): For best results, remove the rollers but wait until your hair has cooled before you comb it out.

- Curling iron: Plug it in, wrap your hair around the wand, and wait a minute. When you unroll—you've got curls. The wands come in superfat models that produce the most natural-looking curls.

Blow-dryers

They curl, straighten, style, and can also dry out your hair something fierce—so never hold them too close. They come in every color and shape, but here are the important things to look for:

- High wattage: Most dryers range from 1,200 to 1,875 watts. Choose one with at least 1,500 watts, but buy one with higher wattage if you need to straighten your curly hair.

- Three settings: High for thick, coarse hair, medium for medium hair, and low for very fine hair.

- A cool-off button: Finish your hair styling with a blast of cool air to help set and seal it.

- Attachments: **Nozzle** to direct the air, **volumizer** to lift the hair away from the roots, creating maximum body, and **diffuser** to soften and spread out the air flow so it doesn't frizz up your curly hair.

My favorite blow-dryer is Supersolano's 1600 red and black model.

The Indispensable Tool?

Scotch tape: no tool quite like it. Tape wet bangs or strange cowlicks in place until they dry.

Natural Products

There are a number of products you can whip up that are totally natural and free of additives, preservatives, and chemicals—except for my recipe for avocado mash. You can store most of them for up to two weeks (if they don't contain food products like yogurt or avocado). It's possible to drive a guy wild with the scent of vanilla.

Natural Color

For blondes, the tried and true lemonade fix: Spray the juice from two lemons on thoroughly wet hair, particularly around the hairline. If possible, sit in the sun for half an hour, then rinse. If the sun isn't an option, mix the lemon juice with conditioner and work through your hair. Rinse after fifteen minutes. This natural hair lightener makes hair glow, but it isn't recommended if you have very dry hair because lemon is astringent and will dry hair even more.

For brown hair and redheads: Make a pot of strong chamomile tea, let it cool, and work it into your wet hair. Blow-dry for a sunny, cinnamony glow.

For black or very dark brown hair, *only* if your hair is not oily: Take used coffee grinds and mix with a teaspoon of olive oil and two teaspoons of sour cream or vanilla yogurt. Work the mixture into wet hair, leave on for twenty minutes, then rinse and blow-dry for a great shine.

Also for very dark hair (it can be oily): Mash a half pint of blueberries and apply to your hair. Cover your hair with a shower cap for twenty minutes, then rinse. Your raven hair will have beautiful highlights.

Herbal Shampoos

Clarifying chamomile shampoo

4 chamomile tea bags
1½ cups water
4 tablespoons of pure soap flakes (Ivory is good)
¼ tablespoon of glycerine (find in any health food store)

Steep the tea bags in 1½ cups boiled water for ten minutes. Remove the tea bags, add soap flakes, and let stand until soap is soft. Blend in the glycerine. Use weekly on wet hair. Pour into a bottle with a cap and store in a dark, cool place.

Botanical herbal shampoo

¼ cup herbs or dried flowers (try rosemary,
    spearmint, peppermint, sage, marjoram, orange
    blossoms, dandelion, or comfrey root)
1 cup water
1 teaspoon liquid castile soap
1 teaspoon apricot kernel oil or vanilla or almond extract
2 drops essential oil, an undiluted pure oil extracted
    directly from plants or flowers: Choose the fragrance
    you like from any health food store.

Put the dried herbs or flowers in a heatproof bowl. Boil the water; pour over the herbs. Let steep for about twenty minutes. Pour the water through a strainer set over another bowl. Remove strainer, then stir in the castile soap, the apricot oil, or the vanilla or almond extract, and the essential oil. Pour into a bottle with a cap. Use once a week. Store bottle in a dark place.

Natural Conditioners

Olive oil is the trendy new ingredient in many hand lotions and face washes. I've been telling my clients to try olive oil as a deep-conditioning hair treatment if their hair is not naturally oily. Massage a quarter-sized dollop (less for short hair) into your hair and scalp, leave on for an hour, then rinse with warm water, then as-cold-as-you-can-take-it water.

Try my honey-love rinse for superb shine for any hair. Add a teaspoon of honey to four cups of hot water and mix well. After shampooing, apply the mixture to your hair, leave in about three minutes, then rinse.

This avocado mash adds shine to everything *but* oily hair (make just enough for one treatment—don't store it). Take a ripe avocado, cut it in half, and remove the pit. Scoop out the meat from one half and mash in a bowl. Add three tablespoons of your regular conditioner. Mix well and apply to hair; leave on for seven to ten minutes. Rinse very well. What shine! What softness!

A Smashing Fragrant Spray

Here's a recipe for a fragrant spray that's great for any hair but particularly for curly hair. Lavender is a great cleansing agent and its fragrance is wonderful. A quick spritz revives your curls; finger-scrunch them after spritzing. Add four drops of pure lavender essential oil to one quart of bottled water. Make a big batch, fill a small travel-size spray bottle, and store the rest.

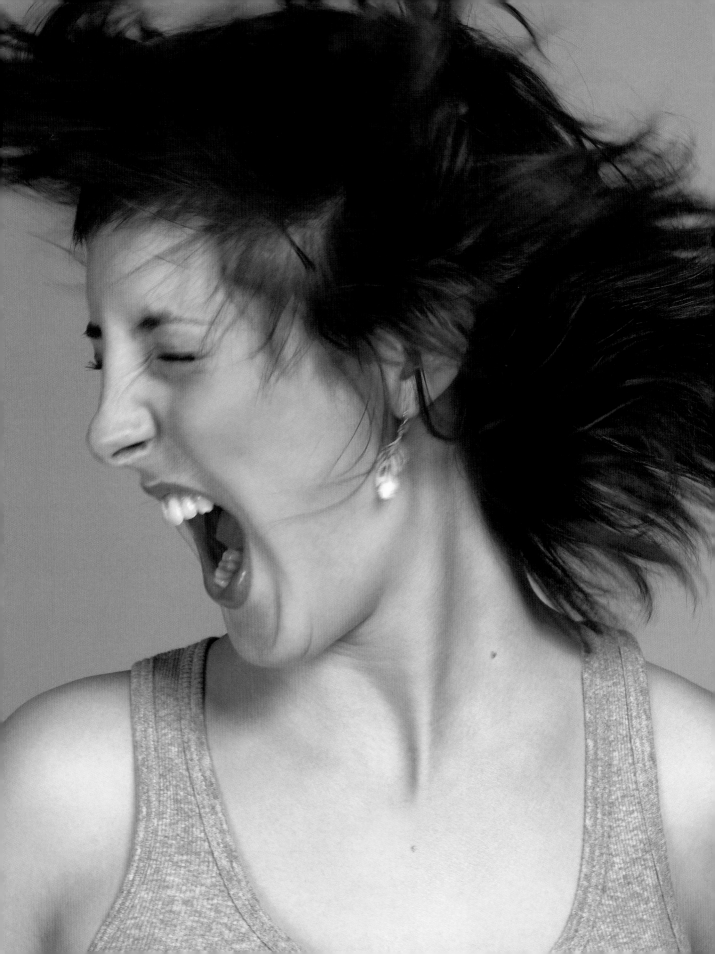

Cut and Color | 4

We've covered the first two elements of finding the best hairstyle for your individual hair. First, we've identified your hair texture and you've learned what options you have to change the texture if you're not happy with your appearance. Second, we've covered hair care for your individual kind of hair. Now comes the cut.

To find the best cut for your hair texture and the shape of your face, you need professional help. Your style will hold only if the cut holds, and the cut will hold only if it's right for your hair texture. It takes training and experience to give a great cut. Fool around with temporary color and with different styling products by yourself, but, please, even if you've never been to a hairdresser for a cut, this is the time to do it. Discuss the cut that's perfect for the texture of your hair, your face, and your body shape, with the stylist.

How to Talk to Your Hairstylist

Sometimes, a teenager sits in my chair and she's absolutely tongue-tied. The same girl that had so much to say to her best friend hours before hasn't a word to say to me. I wonder why.

I suspect it's because most of you think an expert should just *know stuff*—and I should automatically know the best way to do your hair. Well, I do know a lot about hair and how *I'd* like to see it—but what I don't know is what you envision, realistic or not. It's you who has to wear that hairdo. A new hairstyle is a collaboration between the hairstylist, Mother Nature, and, most important, the client. This is no time to be shy. A good stylist depends on you to share your thoughts.

Seventeen-year-old
Eva Amurri.

When you sit in any stylist's chair for a haircut, a professional needs to look at and touch your hair before it's washed to see how it falls naturally.

Then, you need to tell your stylist

- how short (or long) you want your hair to be

- how much time you want to spend doing your hair

- what kind of style you think you want—bangs or no bangs, part or no part

- what drives you nuts about caring for your hair

A Picture Is Worth a Thousand Words

It is a help if you bring along some pictures of the style you love.

We both know you're not going to look like Jennifer Aniston or Mandy Moore or whoever is wearing the hairstyle in the photograph, but a photograph gives us a springboard to start talking and thinking about what would look fabulous on you. If you're planning to make some color changes, a photograph is the only way for me to understand what you mean when you say, for example, "*I want to be a sunny blonde*." One person's idea of *sunny blond* may be my idea of *honey blond*. A photograph of what you want is the only way to get our signals straight.

Your hairstylist may offer some suggestions, which you may take or disregard. It's your choice. But talk to your hairstylist. Be open and consider the expert's suggestions. Then make up your own mind.

Stop for a Minute

Before you take the big step—and a haircut is always a major step—think about the following.

What Does Your Hair *Want* to Do?

Straight hair wants to fall straight. You may curl it temporarily—and it's fun to go against type for a while—but in the end, your best style will be straight hair—falling like a waterfall. But, there's more to it than that. If your hair is straight and not too thick, it should be layered instead of bluntly cut. If it's very straight and very thick, consider a soft, just-at-the-roots permanent to give its straightness better form. If it's straight and very fine and thick, go with a blunt,

Pardis shows me the style she likes.

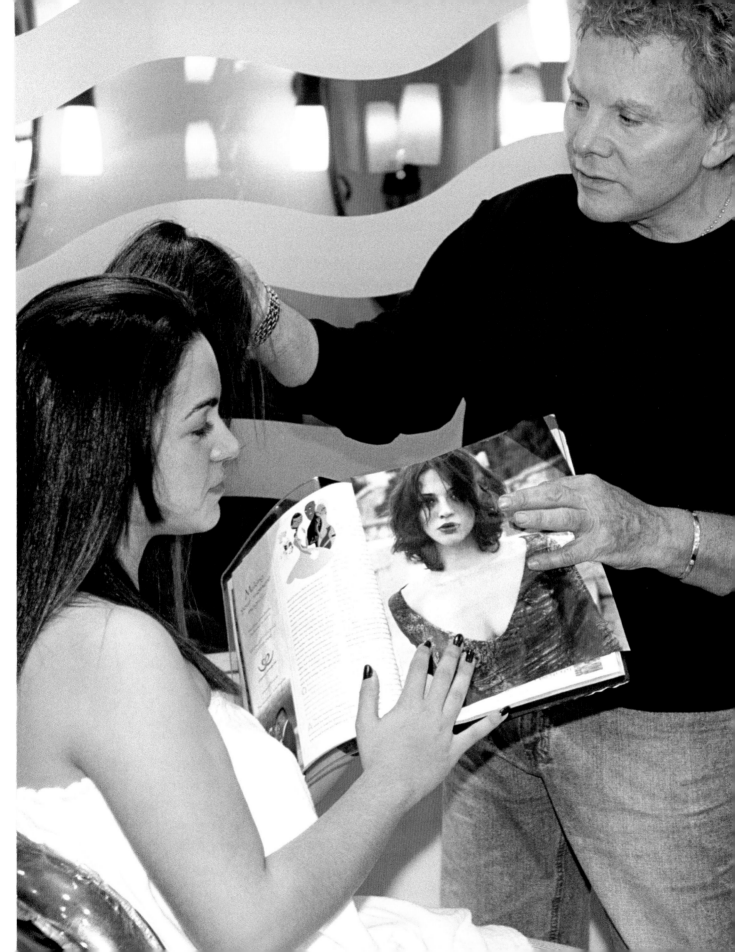

Round

Does your face show more cheeks than cheekbones?
Do you have a wide, full chin?

*Your face is round, like Mandy Moore's or
even Kelly Osbourne's.*

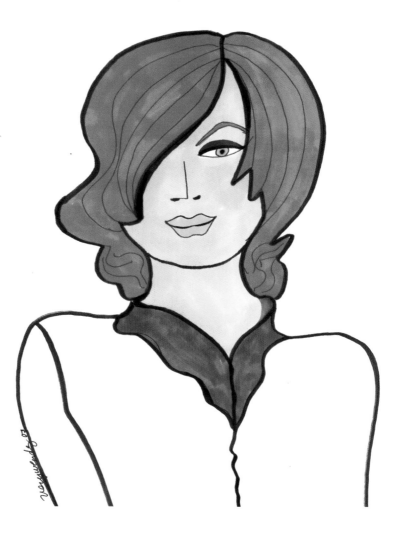

Best style: long (at least shoulder-length), layered, layered, layered hair—with more height on top to "ovalize" the roundness. You might also try a short, feathered, fringy cut that's brushed toward the face—a very narrowing and sophisticated effect. Grow in the bangs but adopt some wisps to soften the roundness. A side part will appear to make your face longer.

Avoid very curly, very full hair.

Long and Narrow

Is your face long, your chin thin and narrow?

You have a long, narrow face, like Brandy's, Jennifer Love Hewitt's, and Jamie Lee Curtis's.

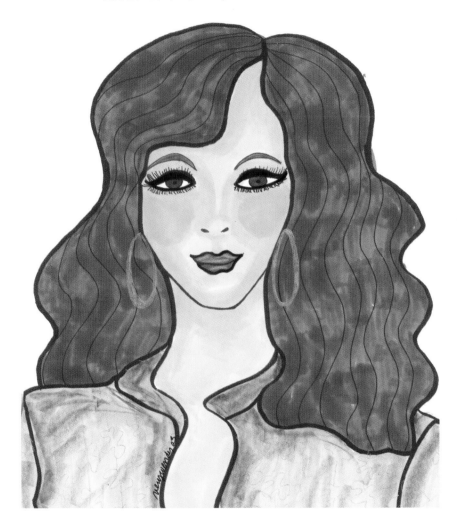

Best style: a cut that doesn't make your hair full or high at the top of your head. You need to neutralize and shorten the longness with fullness around the face. Hair that's cut above chin length makes your face look even narrower. If your hair isn't naturally curly, consider a permanent to best achieve a fuller look. A side part widens the forehead and neutralizes the length. If you like them, wisps around the face soften an angular face.

Avoid long, all-one-length cuts.

Oval

Is your face more oval than square, round, or long?

You're a lucky girl—your oval face looks terrific in almost every cut, like Jennifer Aniston's or Iman's.

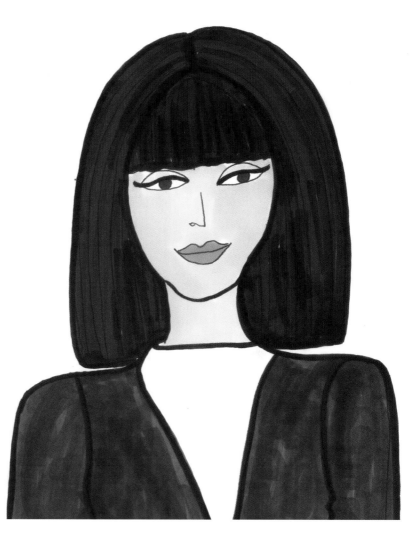

Best style: You can try almost anything if the texture of your hair allows it. I love straight, angled-at-the-jaw cuts for this wonderful face shape. Very curly hair calls out for short and chic, but you also look divine with a mass of long, pre-Raphaelite curls—or the straight, layered look Jennifer Aniston made so popular.

Avoid nothing.

Balancing Your Features with a Good Cut

A well-designed hairstyle can seem to restructure your face. There are simple tricks with which you can experiment. If, for example, you dislike your very broad or very low forehead, instead of blaming your genes, take a practical step and make a change in your hairstyle.

- Hair swept back off the face in a ponytail, chignon, or braid makes a long nose seem shorter.

- Bangs—even wisps of bangs—shorten the face and a high forehead.

- A severe, back-from-the-face style flatters a low forehead.

- A full, rounder, shorter hairstyle works well with a very small face.

- Short hair curling onto the face below the cheekbone softens a powerful jawline.

- A pointy chin calls out for hair width at the jawline; very short hair only emphasizes the chin.

- Hair cut just below chin level balances a receding chin. Lots of waves or curls also distract from this feature.

- Bangs, or even wisps of bangs, disguise an uneven hairline.

- Large eyeglasses can spoil the look of a neat, feathery haircut, and very thin frames can be overpowered by big hair. Take your eyeglasses to the salon when having a haircut so your stylist can take them into consideration when deciding on a style.

What Cut Works for Your Hair Texture?

Straight, Coarse, and Thick

Try a layered, long look for a liquid flow.
Avoid a blunt, all-one-length cut—it will stand shapelessly away from your pretty face.

Straight, Coarse, and Thin

Try a blunt, all-one-length cut on shorter hair to make that hair *move*.
Avoid layering, which will make it look a tad bushy. If your hair's already layered, try a gentle root perm for controlled volume.

Straight, Fine, and Thick

Try a blunt, chin-length cut with a little bit of fine layering on the top and around the sides to frame the face and give some movement.

Avoid any tool or cutting process (sometimes called texturizing) that might thin the hair—like using a razor that cuts into the hair layers. A scissors always gives more control.

Straight, Fine, and Thin

Try a short, blunt cut to give volume and perhaps a mild perm to give fullness.

Avoid long hair at all costs. Length will pull down your hair and make it look thinner and wispier.

Straight, Medium, and Thick

Try shorter layers for volume. It will also look great layered to your shoulder. You might try a perm on just the underneath layer to give body to the hair and yet keep the sleek, straight look.

Avoid nothing. You have the hair that makes men weep! Try everything that appeals to you.

Straight, Medium, and Thin

Try a soft, blunt bob around chin length. I call it the *Chanel* cut, after the famous designer. Hair should ideally be parted on the side. There's not much lift—it's a flatter look. But you might also choose to taper just the ends of the hair to achieve a gentle flip.

Avoid any style longer than shoulder-length. Also avoid permanents; better to keep to a smooth, sleek, shining line.

Curly, Coarse, and Thick

Try a shortish, cropped, layered cut (cut with the natural curl, not against it). If you can carry it off, this hair also looks great in a big, wild (but layered) mane.

Avoid a blunt cut. It won't last for ten minutes. If you're having highlights applied, avoid the flat iron.

Curly, Coarse, and Thin

Try lots of cut texturizing (cutting into the hair on an angle to make layers), but the stylist should not use a thinning scissors or razor, which make the hair frizzy. A sharp scissors should be used or else your hair will stick out like an umbrella.
Avoid blunt cuts.

Curly, Fine, and Thick

Try a blunt, chin-length cut. Since your hair is thick, you don't need the volume you'd get from layering.
Avoid shoulder-length hair. If fine hair is allowed to grow long, it can look wispy.

Curly, Fine, and Thin

Try a layered and stacked cut. If you use a diffuser on your blow-dryer, your own natural curl will provide the volume.
Avoid straight, blunt cuts.

Curly, Medium, and Thick

Try almost anything. You look great in long or short hair because of your hair's natural body. You can even do a wedge cut like skater Dorothy Hamill's. Lots of framing around the face also looks wonderful. Bangs look super.
Avoid nothing. You have beautifully workable hair.

Curly, Medium, and Thin

Try a long, precision blunt cut. Straight-across bangs are also fine for you.
Avoid short hair cut all one length—your hair will lie flat. Go with the layers.

Frizzy Hair

Try a short, cropped style like Halle Berry's.
Avoid long, blunt cuts—they just won't work.

Color

At last, we come to the final part of my equation—color.

I used to think you should be over eighteen to change the color of your hair, but now with the new, safe, temporary colors, I love to see a teen experimenting. It's good for your psyche. Here's the wonderful part: Unlike cutting hair, you can do it yourself and do it well.

We live in a new world of color—and while it's fun to choose a funky color for a wild mood (see Kelly Osbourne with her royal blue/pink/whatever chunks), you can also explore the world of subtle highlights, glowing lowlights, or delicate frosting, all of which I will explain. The beauty of color is that it either washes out or grows out. With the temporary wash-out color rinses now available, or with the marvelously campy color additions you can just attach or paint on in no time, you can be blond for a week or raven haired for the prom. You can spike your hair purple, red, or green just for the heck of it. You can even use mascara or spray paint on your hair, or paint only the tips really light or dark (you can cut them off if you decide you hate it).

My opinion? I love temporary color rather than permanent color for girls in their teens. They're mood lighteners, and they don't contain ammonia or peroxide. You don't have to keep them for more than a few hours if you've made a terrible blunder, and you can even redye sections in other colors for another version of you. You will have plenty of time for serious color changes as you grow older. Enjoy your natural color and spike it with changing shades as the mood takes you.

Some Words About Serious Color

If you do decide to go for permanent color, you should be familiar with the hair color language. Before you decide on permanent color (which won't wash out— you have to wait until it grows out), you must consider whether you have:

- the skin tone for the color you want. If, for example, you're going for soft and pretty, the fairest of skin will look harsh with inky-black hair, although it might be interesting for your "witch-week" look. Don't choose the color you want without consulting your own complexion.

- the time and money for the color. You can play with fun, temporary color, but if you want to change your color permanently, do you have

Color Smarts

- Adding color to your hair makes the hair shaft swell, so very fine hair looks thicker and fuller.

- Adding highlights and lowlights makes very thick hair more supple and manageable.

- If you have very thin hair, you don't want to bleach it too light; it will make your hair look even thinner.

- Before going swimming in chlorinated water with color-treated hair, put a layer of the thickest, most inexpensive conditioner over your hair to provide a chlorine shield. I like a product called Queen Helene conditioner. Rinse thoroughly afterward—it's pretty gloppy.

the *time* to be a double-process blonde? Frequent trips to a professional would be necessary and the cost could be prohibitive.

Okay, you've decided you're going all the way with permanent color, and for this, you want natural-looking color that will complement your skin tones—this is not the time for the purple braids. It's important that you don't do any wild experimentation here, because this color is *you,* for as long as it takes to grow out. And hair grows about a half inch a month—you do the math.

Now, check out the following hair coloring terms, deconstructed:

Permanent color: It's not really permanent, as in forever, but it does last until new hair growth arrives—or you cut it off. The new hair growth is commonly known as "roots"—as in, "God, my roots are an inch long, I must get my hair done!" You cannot apply permanent color to your hair by yourself: the chemicals used are too strong and too tricky for anyone but a professional to work with.

Semipermanent color: usually rinses out in four to six shampoos. Some semipermanent colors last from eighteen to twenty-four shampoos. Read the instructions to see how long you have to be purple-haired.

Highlights: gentle veins of lighter color created by bleach applied to sections of your hair. You have to wait for highlights to grow out to make them go away. Blondes look great with silvery highlights; darker hair looks best with coppery or reddish lights—never blond. Highlights can be applied in delicate, thin bands or in chunks, which are very popular today.

Lowlights: gentle, and usually darker-than-your-natural-color streaks. Many shades are possible, including strawberry blond or red.

Tips: lightening *some* ends of your hair.

Single-process color: Only one application of color is placed on the hair, or on the roots of previously colored hair, for about thirty minutes. If your hair is bleached from the sun, ask your hairdresser to comb the color through your hair for the last three minutes.

Double-process color: a radical change in the color of your hair from dark to light. First, your natural hair color is bleached out, then the new color is applied. Double-process color needs frequent touch-ups.

Tinfoil process: Color (for lowlights) or bleach (for lightening) is applied to small sections of hair, and then these are wrapped in squares of foil to separate them from the rest of the hair.

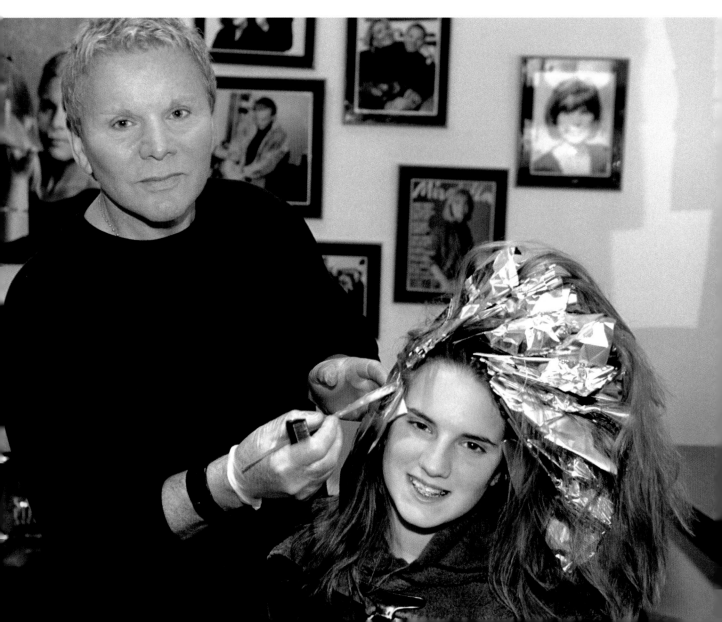

Henna: a natural vegetable dye and also a great shine *reducer.* Don't ask me for henna—I never work with it anymore. Too unreliable.

Mood Color

This is hair color that's custom-made for mercurial moods! You can test a shade, then get rid of the color, *almost* as fast as the mood passes. Mood colors come in:

Semipermanent color: These fairly new coloring products come in gels, hair mascaras, pomades, sprays, creams, rinses, color by paintbrush—almost every variety of packing. They change color, soften color, or make the color of your own hair more intense. Semipermanent color can be used to widen or narrow face shapes. It can add highlights, lowlights, or insane streaks for fun, and it all washes away eventually—in from seven to twenty-eight shampoos. In some cases, you'll thank your lucky stars this is true. In other cases, you'll *love* the difference.

Temporary color: This doesn't really change your hair color but mostly tones or boosts your own shade. It washes away in about four to fourteen shampoos. There's a red flag here. Temporary color has been known to ooze off even before you hit the shampoo. "It's not easy being green."

Glimmer and glitter: Sometimes you don't need real color to achieve a whole new look. Glitter gives glints and twinkles of color—great for a special event. Try it just in your part for fun.

Do-It-Yourself Color Products

These products are available in many hair supply stores, and perhaps your hairdresser carries some. Be sure to follow the individual directions.

Important: Many hair color products warn you to keep the color away from your eyes. Being careless can cause eye damage and even, in some cases, blindness.

Semipermanent Color Products

Cream Pots

Little pots of colors with names like Spring Green, Plum, and Lagoon Blue are put out by a company called *Tish & Snooky's Manic Panic* ("*Live fast and dye your hair*" is its motto). The directions say it works best on hair prelight-

Molly in foil.

ened to very blond, but some of the colors may give highlights to darker hair. The color fades gradually with each shampoo.

Birthday Cake Color

Jazzing, a nice product put out by Clairol, comes in a plastic bottle with a pointed applicator that looks exactly like the tube with which you write on birthday cakes. *Jazzing* can be applied to be either *very temporary* color (leave it on for five to ten minutes, rinse, and shampoo) or *longer-lasting, semipermanent color* (leave it on for up to thirty minutes, put on a plastic cap, and process with heat before you shampoo). Read the instructions for exact directions. It comes in a rainbow of colors like Bold Gold or Cherry Cola (more cherry than cola). The very temporary color will be gone in just two to five shampoos if you change your mind, and the semipermanent application will last through at least two weeks of daily shampoos.

Nursery School Color

A longer-lasting (from five to forty washes), semipermanent color that really works is called *Punky Colour Cream* and is put out by a company called Jerome Russell. In colors like Apple Green, Plum, and Lagoon Blue, this product works best on already-colored or chemically-treated hair. *Punky* gives a highlighted effect when used on darker hair.

Hair Mascara

This is actually hair paint. I love a product put out by Fiske Industries called *Hair Mascara*. It comes in a tube that looks exactly like a mascara wand except it's used to color hair, not eyelashes. In colors with unimaginative names like Gold, Dark Blue, and Burgundy, *Hair Mascara* is nevertheless great fun for experimenting and it shampoos out easily. The directions for short hair tell you to apply the color in short strokes, but if your hair is long you need to hold a strand and apply the color from root to end. Then, brush through either short or long hair for an instant transformation.

If It Doesn't Glitter, It Doesn't Count

Hair glitter can definitely lend snap, dash, and cool to your hairstyle. I certainly wouldn't recommend it as daily seasoning, but it's fun if you're under

Zemrie with hair mascara.

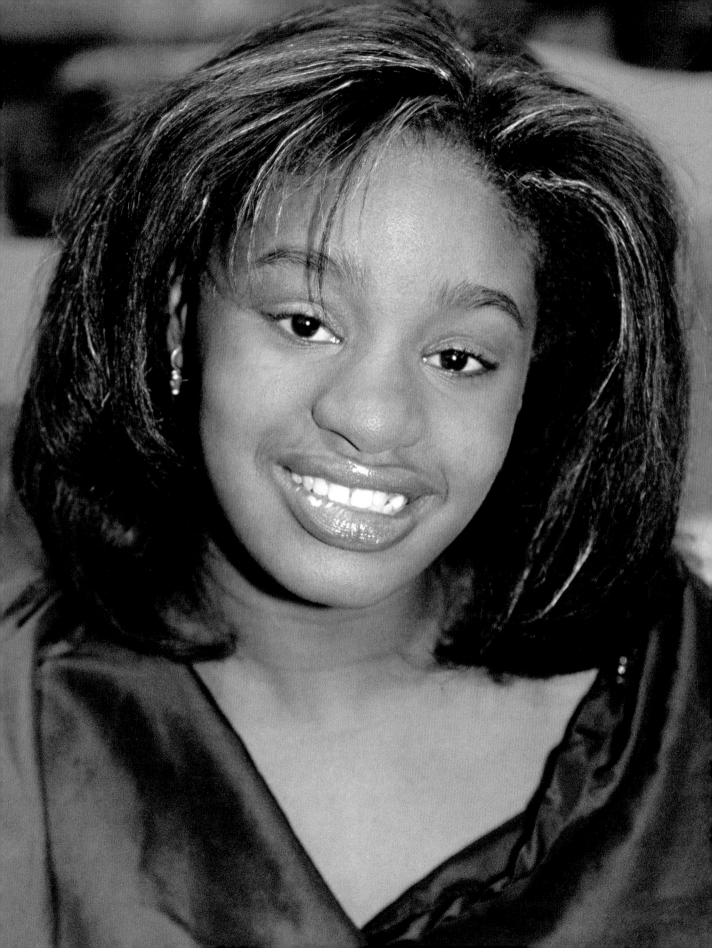

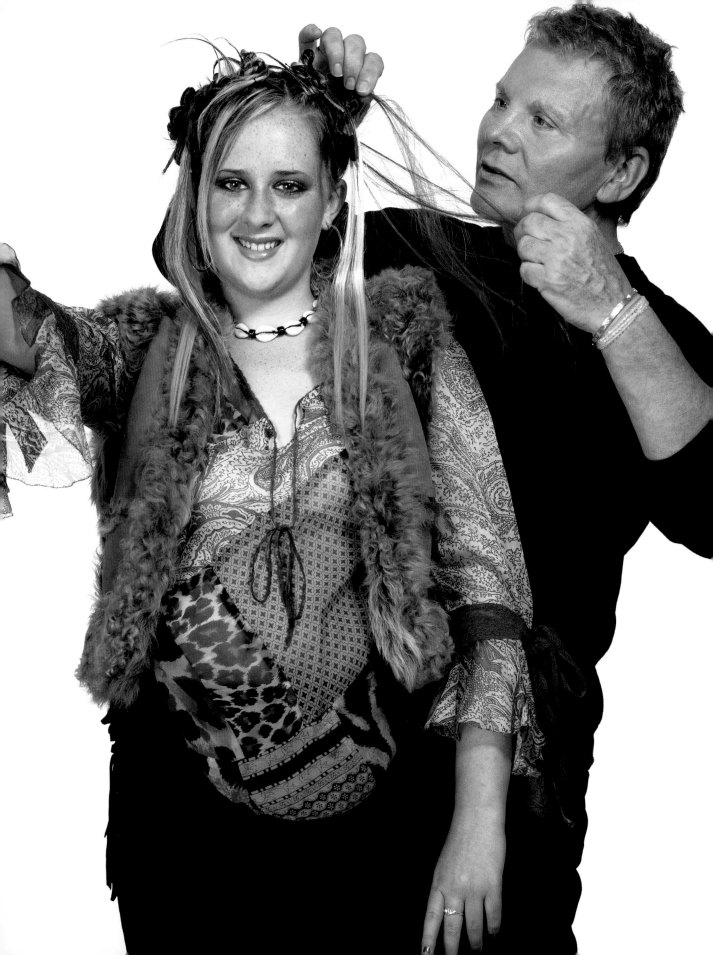

Four Hair Secrets of the Rock Stars

1. **Hair dull?** My show biz clients use a silicone spray for instant sheen (the John Frieda Company puts out a good one or ask your local beauty supply store for its recommendation). Spray it on your brush (not your hair) and lightly move the brush over the hair so as not to disturb your hairdo.

2. **Hair looks granny thin?** Sprinkle some baby powder in your palms, work it into the roots of the hair. Then back comb, with a paddle brush—not a tail comb—section by section, then smooth hair over the back-combed area with a comb.

3. **Hair dirty but no time for a shampoo?** Spray your hands with an aerosol hair spray, massage into hair roots, then brush hair into place.

4. **Hair needs height?** After blow-drying, lift a section of hair where it needs height and spray *underneath* that section—not on top. When you gently place the hair back, it will have more volume and still be glossy and smooth on top.

twenty. One product I like is called *Nasty Girl Glitter Gloss,* which comes in delicious shades like Watermelon. It isn't nasty at all. It's packaged in a small vial attached to a string, and you can wear it around your neck for quick glitter touch-ups when you're feeling the gloomies.

Hair Extensions

If you don't want to color your hair but still long for a kicky look, try a pretty hair extension—sometimes called an addition. (See the how-to illustration on page 66.) You can buy a colorful chignon, ponytail wrap, braids, or simply a long, sleek strip of color on a clip in many hair supply stores. They're often available in your natural hair color, with just a few strands of contrasting color woven in (amethyst? sapphire? emerald?).

Deena.

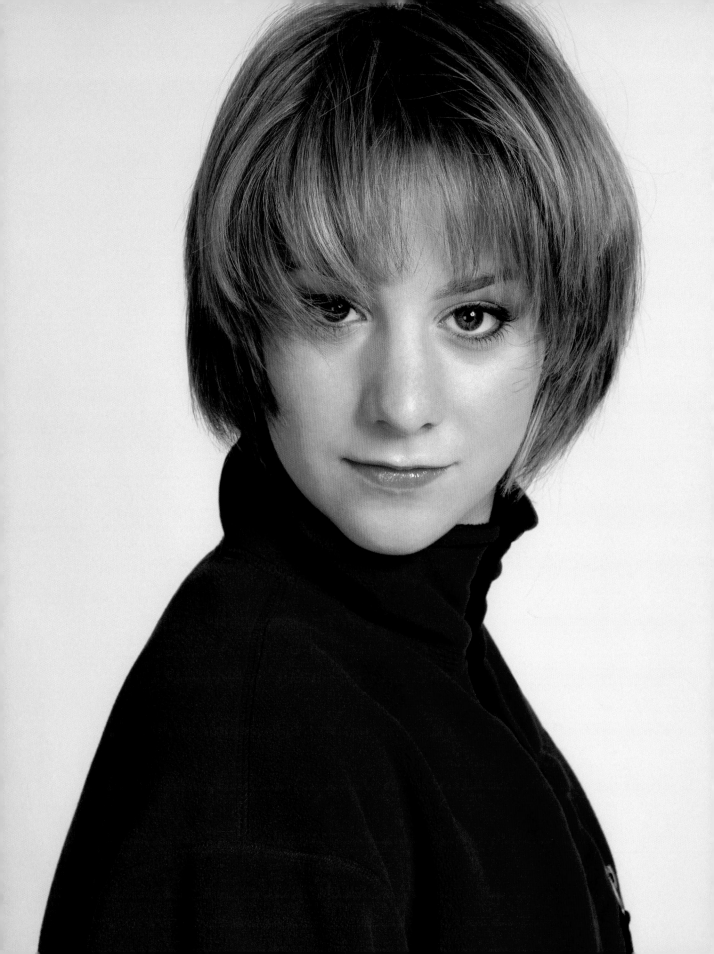

The Elements of Style | 5

Here's the one rule of hair style: If strands escape from your ponytail, if little lumps appear in your French braid, don't despair. The prettiest hair is natural looking, and sweet, loose tendrils make your hairstyle even more appealing. Here are a few classic styles to try:

The Elements of the French Braid

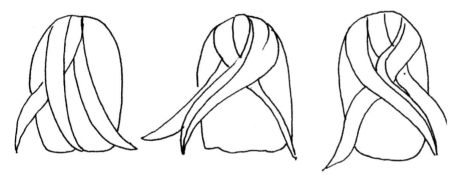

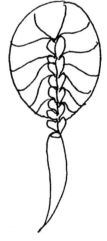

Take a section of your hair from the front of your head, divide it into three even sections, and braid it just one time—not the whole length of the section of hair.

Now comes the French part: Hold the tiny braid you've just made and, with your thumbs, gather about an inch more of hair from each side of the head. Add these to the original strands, then braid the strands just once, again.

Continue like this, picking up more hair as you continue down the braid.

Finish the braid with a covered elastic band, then add a flower or a scrunchie.

Sarah Hughes.

The Elements of the Band Braid

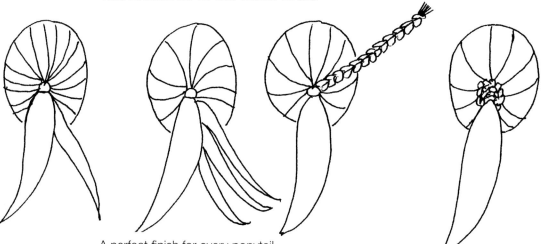

A perfect finish for every ponytail.

Catch almost all your hair into a ponytail, leaving out just a small section near the base of the ponytail.

Put a covered elastic band around the ponytail to hold it in place.

Braid remaining hair into a baby-thin braid.

Wrap the braid around the base of your ponytail, as many times as it will go, covering the elastic.

Secure the braid in place with tiny hair clips. You can use a band braid to finish off a chignon as well. It looks just beautiful.

The Elements of the French Roll

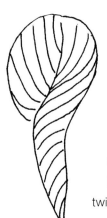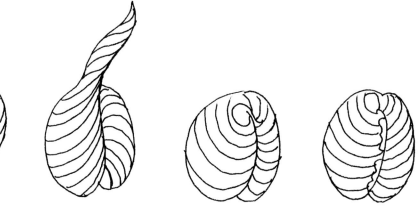

Comb your dampened hair into a ponytail.

Lift up and twist the tail, while holding it taut at the base, and continue twisting up until all hair is coiled.

Circle the ponytail around itself till it forms a spiral.

Fold the end over, tuck it into the base of the ponytail, and secure with hairpins. Add a couple of pretty bone chopsticks for ornaments.

Pull out some side tendrils for a softening effect.

The Elements of Parts

Finding your natural part: After you've towel dried your hair, bend over and shake your head. Flip right side up and you'll see your hair parts naturally on one side or the other or in the middle. Of course, you're not stuck with this part all the time, but choosing your natural part makes hair easier to style because your hair will tend to fall back into its natural swing by midday. When you get a cut, tell the hairdresser where your hair naturally parts.

For variety, check out the following part possibilities:

Zigs: Side parts tend to make long, straight styles fall flat. For extra oomph, height, swing, and volume, add a couple of zigs and zags in the *middle* of your part. With a wide-toothed comb, take tiny sections of hair and switch them back and forth. Gel your fingertips to smooth out stray flyaways.

Middle parts: If you have excellent features, maybe you can swing a straight middle part. Although they seem to flatten out tresses for many, for others, they're stunning—particularly combined with two front baby braids accenting pretty, straight hair.

Side parts: Try a zigzagging side part—it might be very interesting. Or try a short-short side part, which gives volume and some control.

No part at all: Free, loose, unstructured hair often has no part at all. Just sweep it back with your fingers or a brush. You can even clip back the front section of your hair so the no-part hair will hold. Both off-center parts and no parts look wonderful when the hair is swept back to show a pretty face.

Off-center parts: This is a classic part only slightly to the side of center. It's terrific for some faces and gives more volume in front. Try it to see if you like it.

The Elements of Short Hair

You can blow-dry your hair, of course, but a good cut lets you finger dry your hair beautifully—one of my favorite natural looks. After shampooing and conditioning, rub a tiny bit of gel between your hands and work evenly through your hair. Then run your fingers upward and forward through the hair, from root to tip, lifting at the crown to get height. Lift, lift, lift until the hair is reasonably dry. Use your fingertips to flatten and bring the hair in at the nape and, if you wish, behind the ears. The best result is a short, boyish tousle with a rough-and-tumble look.

The Elements of Hair Extensions

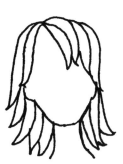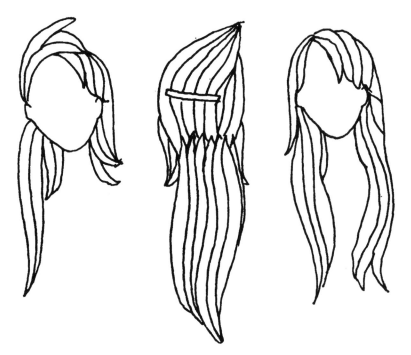

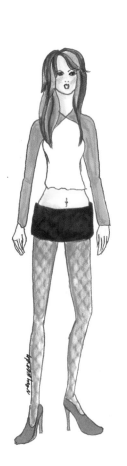

Even if you're not disguising a crummy haircut that's taking forever to grow out, hair extensions can create instant glamour. Just clip up a portion of your back hair; attach the extension with a comb, bobby pins, or clip; and brush your hair over to meld the fake hair with the new waterfall of hair. Hair extensions, incidentally, can lend great volume and interest to short hair.

The Elements of the City Slicker

Another great hair look is the edgy city slicker on Pam at right. With a little gel, brush the sides of your hair behind the ears into a sleek, slicked-down shape—just stunning. If you like, you can leave a few wisps to fall in front of the ears. If your hair is long, the city slicker still works if you pull the hair into a low ponytail, then coil it (and pin it) into a small apple of a chignon.

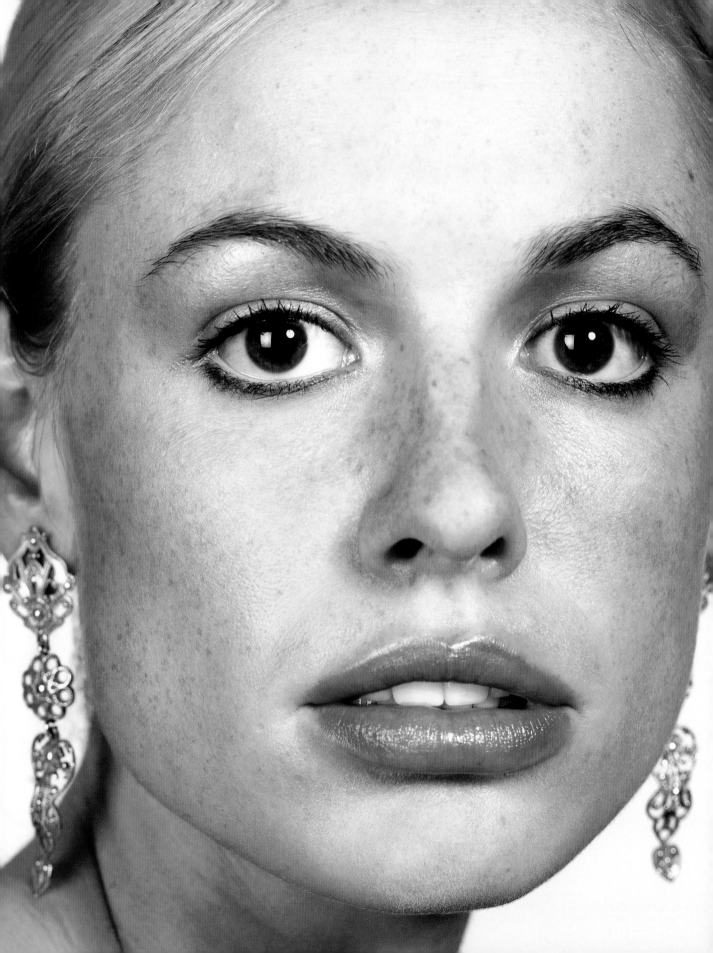

The Elements of Big Hair

It's baaaaaack—though for some teens, especially in Dallas, big hair never left. Here's how to do it:

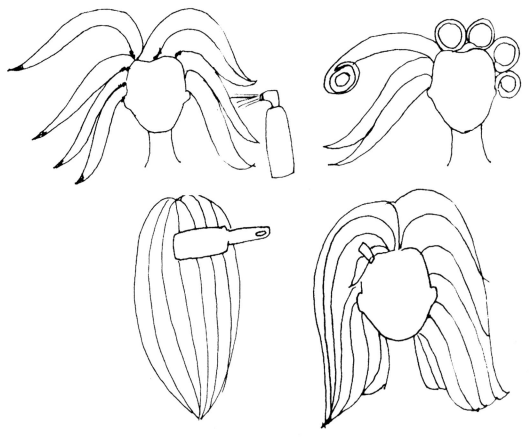

1. Shampoo and condition your hair with products that have thickeners among the ingredients.

2. Dry completely. (If your hair is curly, straighten as you dry.)

3. Rub styling lotion on the roots and ends.

4. Separate hair into two-inch sections and spray (one section at a time) with styling spray.

5. Then, roll the hair onto two-inch hot or Velcro rollers (larger for very wavy or curly hair). If you've used Velcro rollers, heat the rolled hair with your blow-dryer, with the diffuser attached.

6. Remove the rollers and back comb the hair at the roots.

Before: **Here's thirteen-year-old Zemrie, her hair hanging straight and shapeless.**

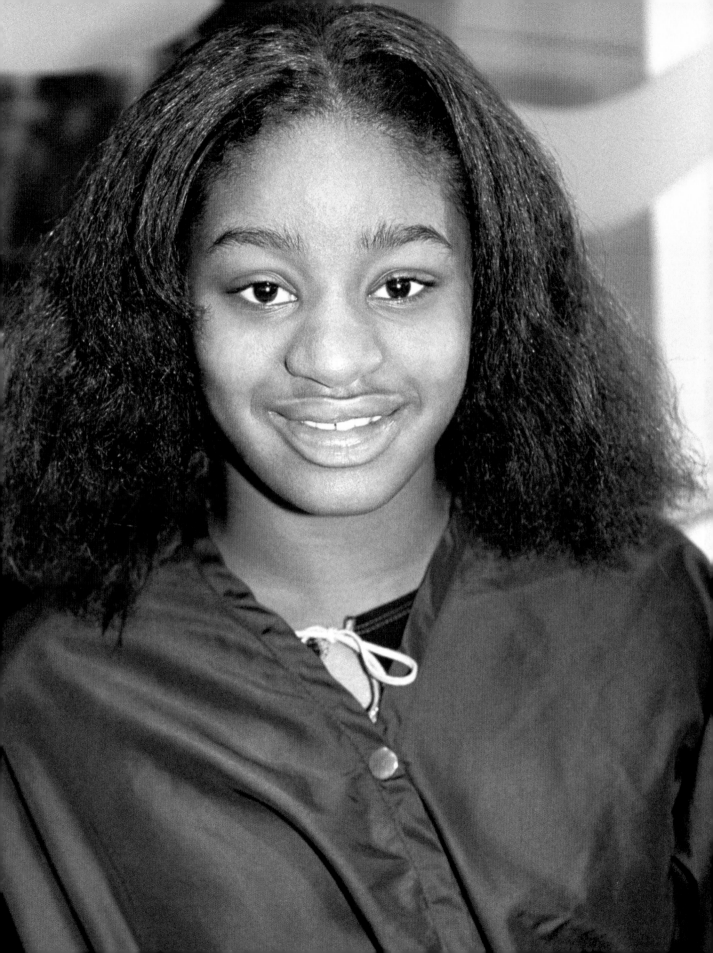

7. Spray your fingers with hair spray—then style.

8. When you're finished, massage a bit of hair pomade or hair wax onto the ends for texture and shine.

The Elements of Bangs

Bangs no longer have to be a straight-across-your-brow fringe. In fact, bangs can instantly change your look and send very direct messages about you. Try:

Shags: Uneven texturizing of your bangs (cutting into them at an angle) is sexy and suggestive. It exaggerates your eyes and says, "I'm feeling romantic." For very curly hair, an antifrizz balm tames and defines the bangs.

Wisps: There's nothing that says *"I'm a risk-taker and pretty daring, also pretty cute"* more than an uneven and eyelash-grazing fringe of wisps. Keep the ends jagged—they should actually look like you cut them yourself. If you want the tips of the wisps to stay defined, use a little silicone gel on the ends. Asymmetrical wisps show another dimension of you.

Streakers: With hair mascara or spray color, streak your bangs with interesting temporary color (red on auburn hair, blue on black hair—you get it). Streakers work well to emphasize your eyes and they minimize a high forehead. The message? Streakers send a message of . . . *unconventional!*

How to Cut Your Own Bangs Without Ruining Your Cool

Trim them dry. Twist your bangs together into one strand and cut the ends in a slight zigzag. Release the hair and trim off any really longer pieces. Bangs are prettier when they're not exactly even.

After: A little makeup and a big-hair blow-dry bestow *excellent* cool. (See Zemrie on page 59—with the hair mascara she requested.)

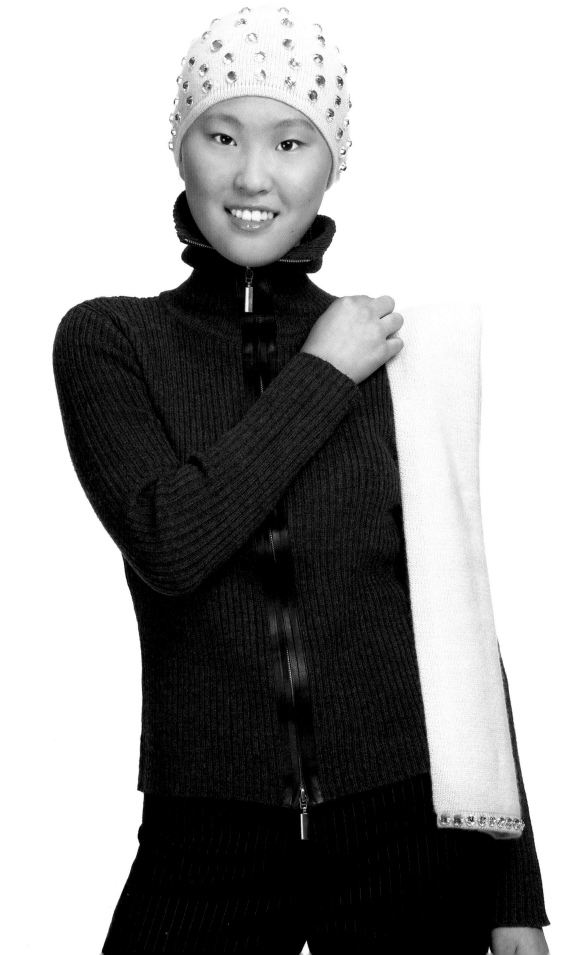

An Adventure: | 6
The New You

I've said you should be you—not J. Lo or Jennifer Aniston—and of course that's true. How can you have a hairstyle that calls for thick, thick hair if yours is baby fine? How can you have long, layered hair if yours is naturally curly and short? Still, this doesn't mean you're utterly stuck with your biology.

On the contrary. You can still make lots of changes—small and large—that will add life, color, and interest to your hair, while staying true to your individual essence. You can invent yourself.

Having great style always depends on imagination added to the working-with-what-you've-got part. You can use these teen years to invent astonishing new possibilities for yourself as long as you pay reasonable attention to the texture of your hair and to what's not possible for you. In fact, you owe it to yourself to experiment. When else are you going to do it—when you're forty-three and a partner in a law firm? This is the *try-it* chapter. Most of the girls who have been photographed for these pages have decided to go for change. That doesn't mean they won't one day go back to their more familiar looks. It just means that for one day, one month, perhaps one year, they're going to try on a different hair look so they can feel adventuresome and new.

You are so over that shaggy bob or that cutesy pixie cut or the hair that drags down your whole face that looked good when you were eight, but now—I don't *think* so. What other look might be waiting out there for you—and how do you accomplish it?

Here are six of the infinite possibilities. There are a zillion other looks you can adapt for your own excellent beauty adventure.

Fourteen-year-old Chisu Yun.

Rita

Half blue/half you: fresh-faced beauty with a million earrings.
Now—blue spiked hair and a tongue stud for good measure (right).

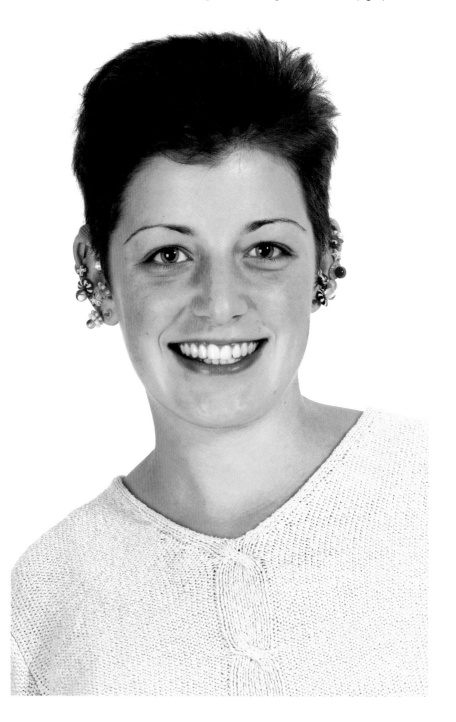

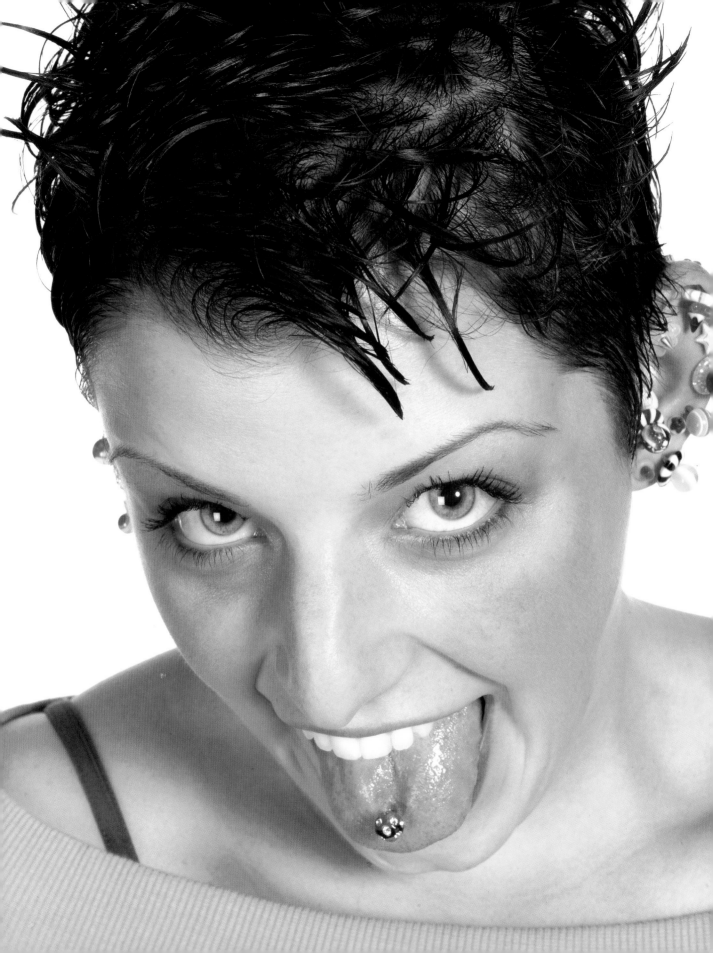

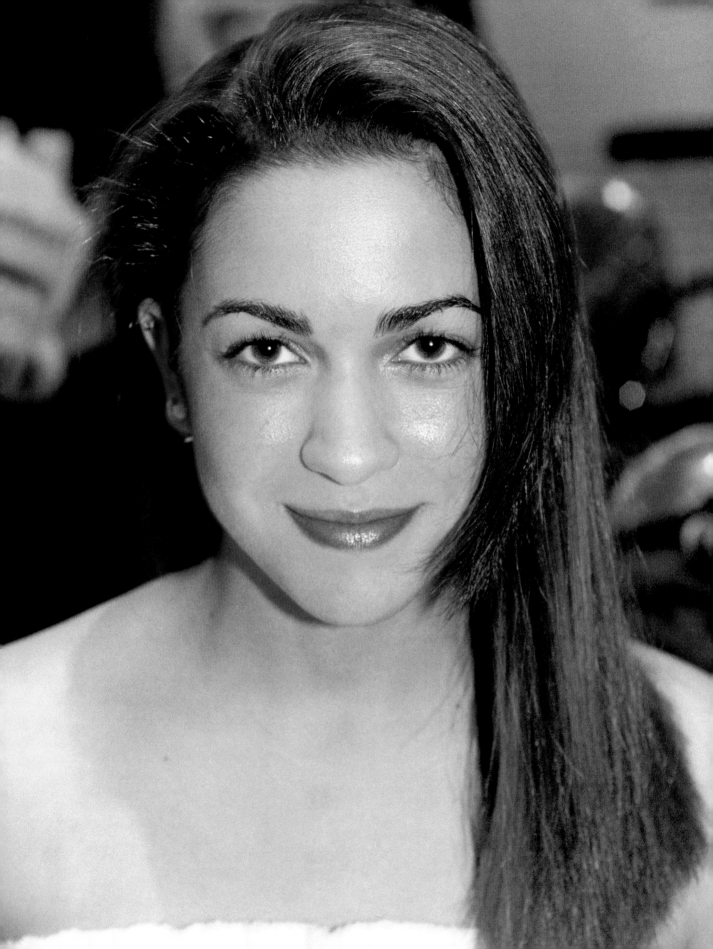

Pardis

I'm a little tired of my curly hair!
Now—straightened and styled long (left).

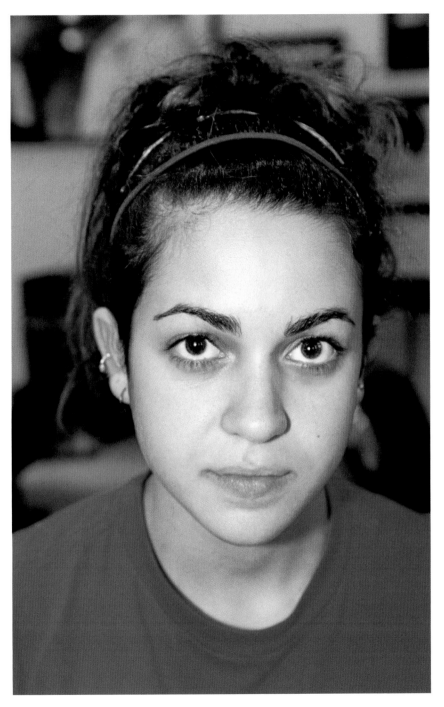

Laura

I love my curly hair! But I need something more!

Now—simply pulled up and back with a giant barrette, lending a new look to this fabulously frizzy hair (right). A few escaping wisps and a little makeup soften an angular face.

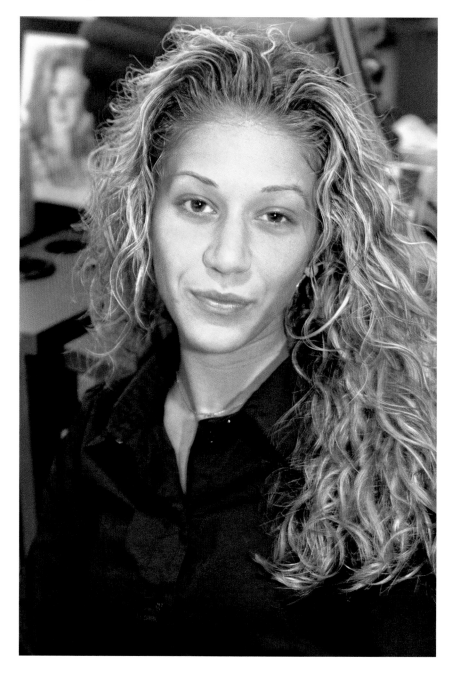

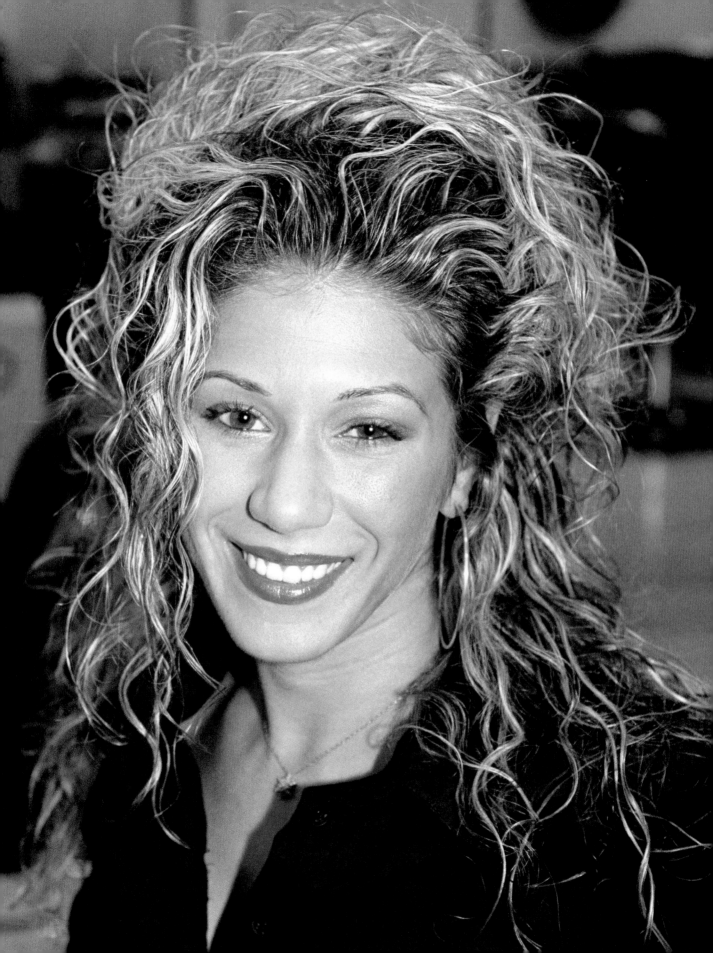

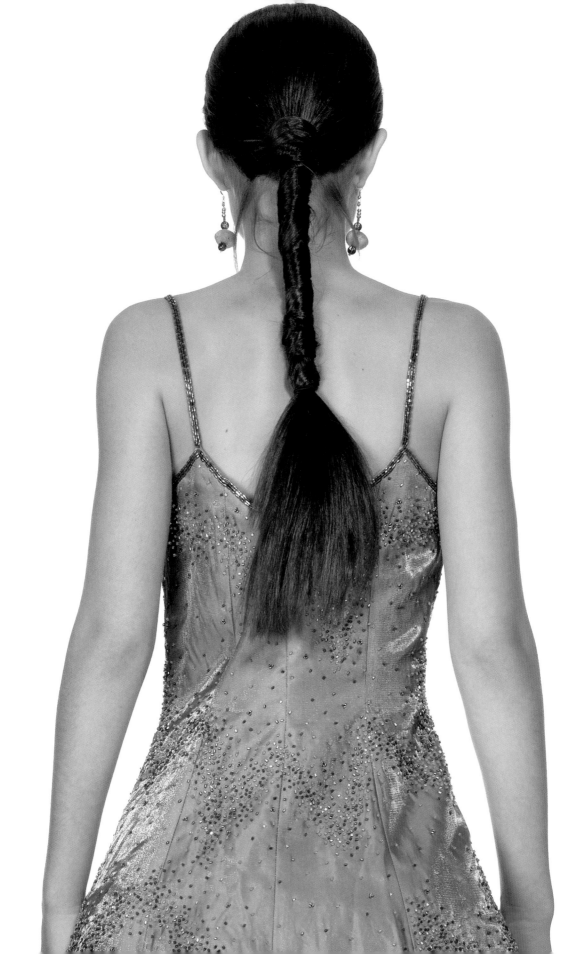

Victoria

A break from my long, loose hair?
Now—a romantic, very low ponytail (left).

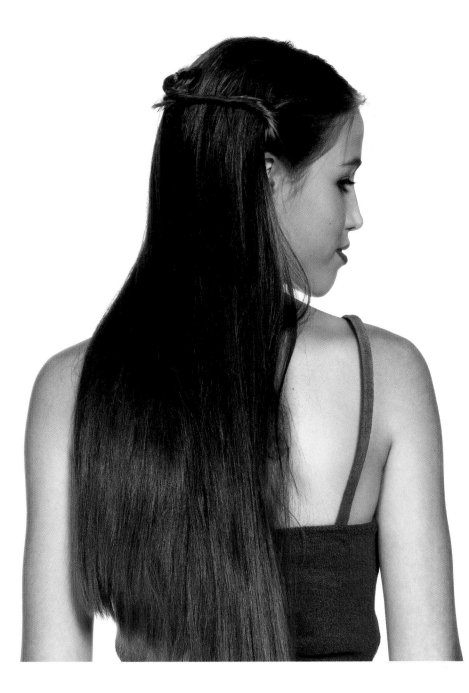

Chisu

I need a new look. Can a fourteen-year-old find high style?
Now—Chisu discovers she has the perfect face for hats! (right).

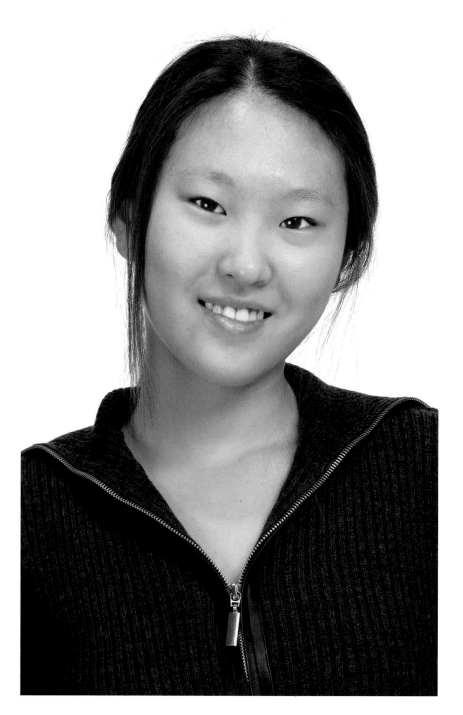

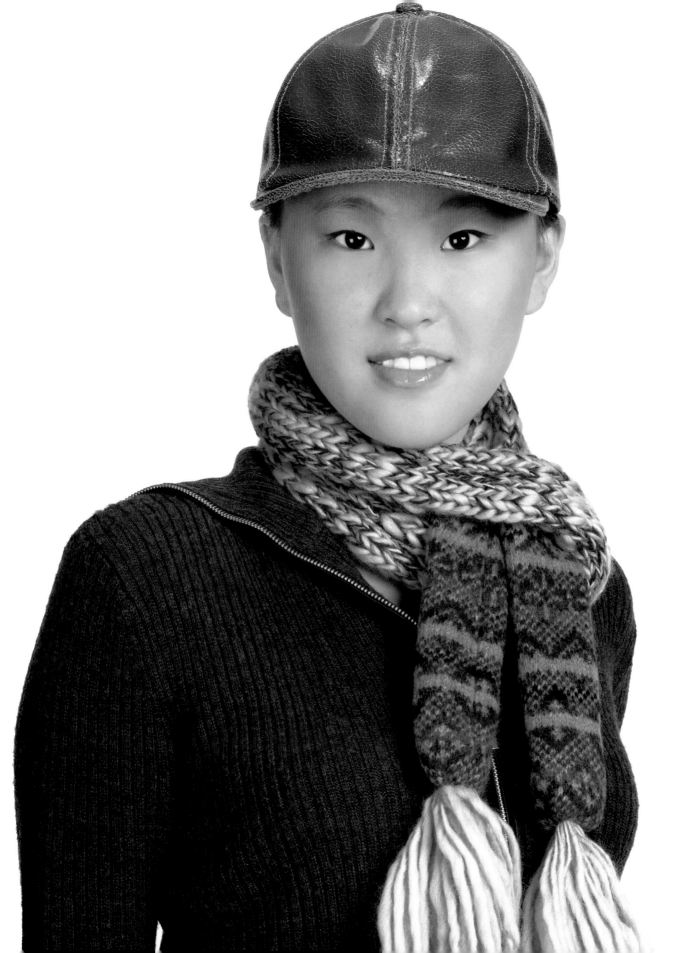

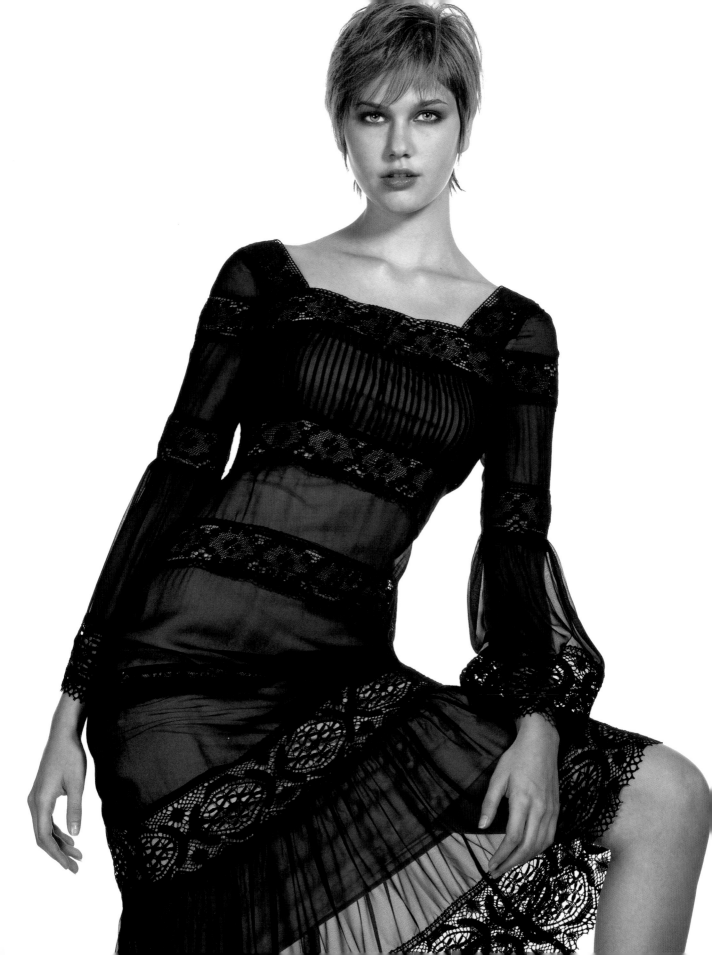

Jennifer

Okay, I'm cute in my Tinker Bell shirt, but I long for sophistication.

Now—Sometimes, it's just a matter of gelling, spiking, and brushing short hair forward . . . and a dynamite dress doesn't hurt (left).

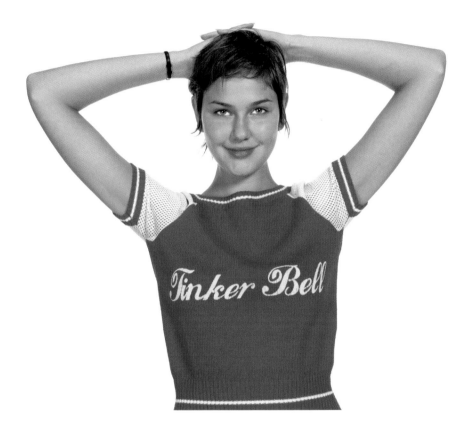

Feel free to combine styles, as you try on a new you. For example, you can take a ponytail and braid it halfway down, then sprinkle glitter in the other half, which you leave in its naturally frizzy state. There are no rules except the ones you make. You're the boss of your hair, and if you choose to be more adventuresome, you'll probably be much admired among your friends.

If your parents are upset when you select a really radical change, it's a good idea to gently explain that nothing is forever. You're just testing limits and they should be happy your most extreme experimentation stops at your hair. Ask them to remember their own teenage years. *Gentle* is the operative word. If you respectfully hear out your parents, chances are they'll object less strenuously.

Don't try to be exactly the same as you were last week or last month. Be new today.

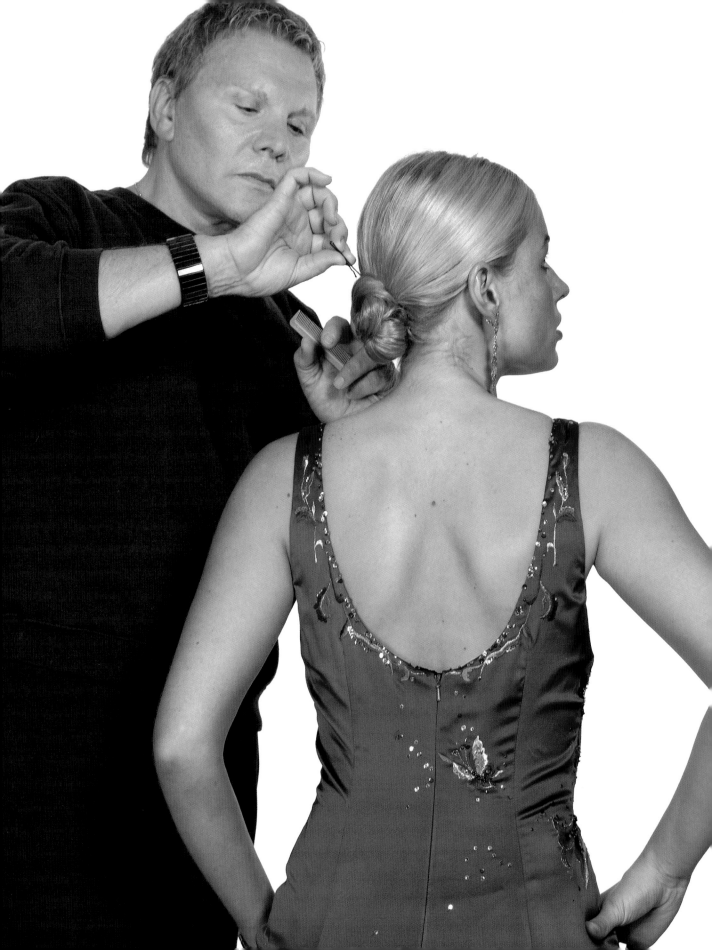

Special Occasion Hair | 7

I know teenagers who never dare to change their look. Whether they go to a rock concert or to a prom, their hair stays the same. This is not fun, in my opinion.

Every occasion is different, and there's no reason why you have to wear the same old hair when you're out with Mr. Right, home with your good friends, or meeting people you want to impress.

Pamela Brown with a chic apple chignon.

Occasions for Which Our Models Wanted New Hair Looks

It's prom night: You want to look— *unforgettable*. You want him to think *flowers, love letters, romance rules*—instead of *basketball is my life*.

Molly, thirteen, goes to school in New York. She's also a budding ballet star and takes dance class daily. Here she is, pre-hair-wash in my salon, getting ready for her close-up.

Baby-braided in front is how she'd wear her hair on prom night with her deep-purple velvet gown. Then, transformed into the girl next door in her pink crocheted separates, Molly simply blow-dries her hair to meet her date for the next night's concert.

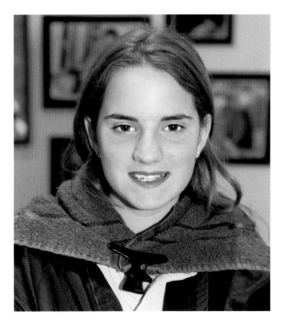

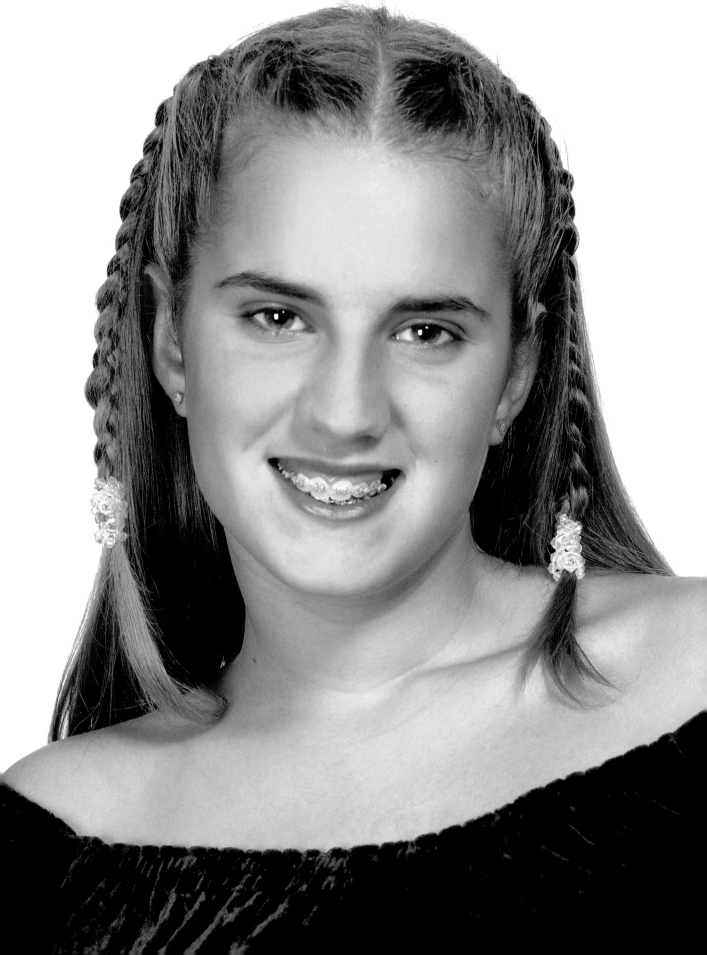

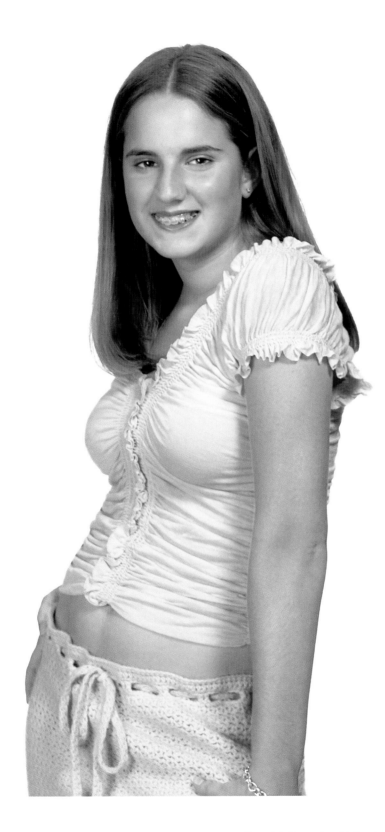

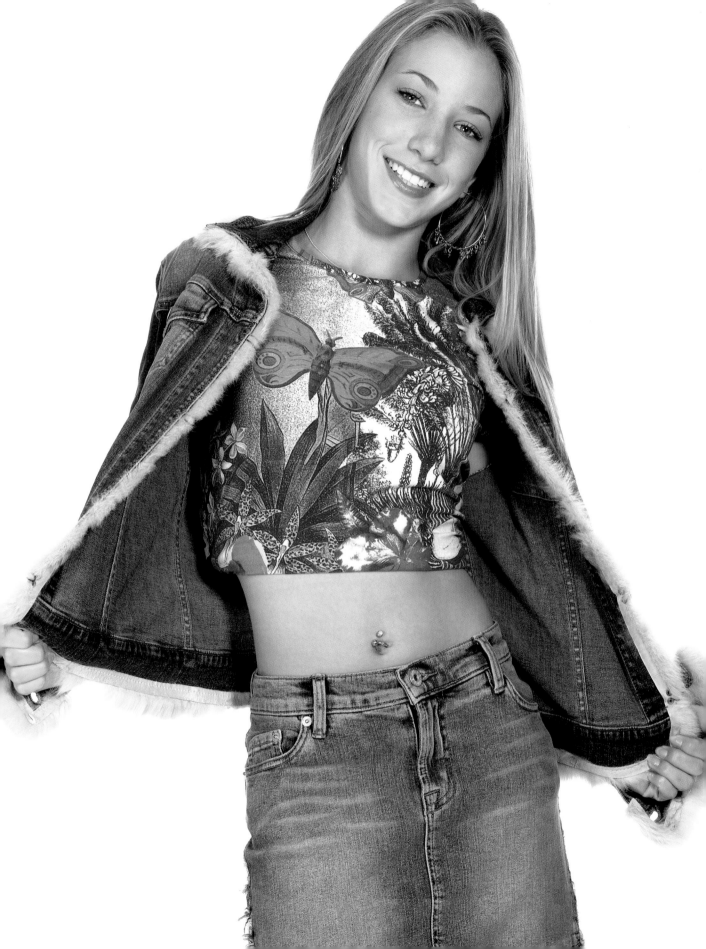

Your friend is fixing you up with her boyfriend's buddy and you want to look hot.

Jenn's a pretty, all-American girl and, being an athlete, hair bunches suit her just fine. But when she wants to look a bit more sophisticated, she irons her beautiful blond hair, dons a midriff-skimming shirt and a trendy jeans jacket and skirt, and she's a pure hottie.

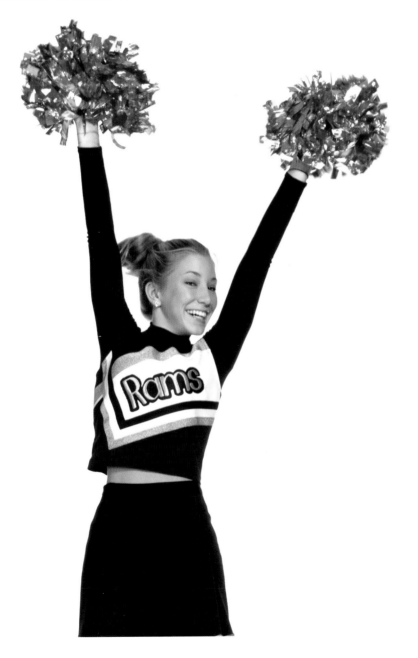

The I-Got-Dumped Haircut: He's dumped you, and you want to make him think *No, no, no—what a blunder, what was I thinking?*

Renee, fifteen, just broke up with her boyfriend. I took one look at her and guessed the truth. Don't ask how—I'm psychic. She says the breakup was agonizing. "I felt used; it made me sad and angry, and I just want him to know what he's missing. That's why I want my hair seriously shorter."

Renee (right), after! It takes a while to get over it, but when you break up with a guy, a new, attention-getting style helps enormously. There's no question—the breakup blues are less indigo when you feel fresh and new—and he sees what he's missing.

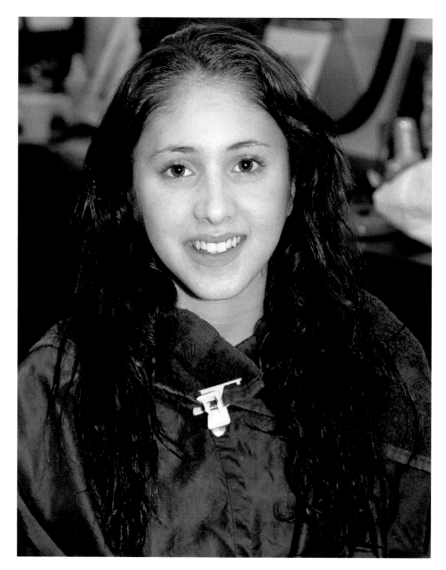

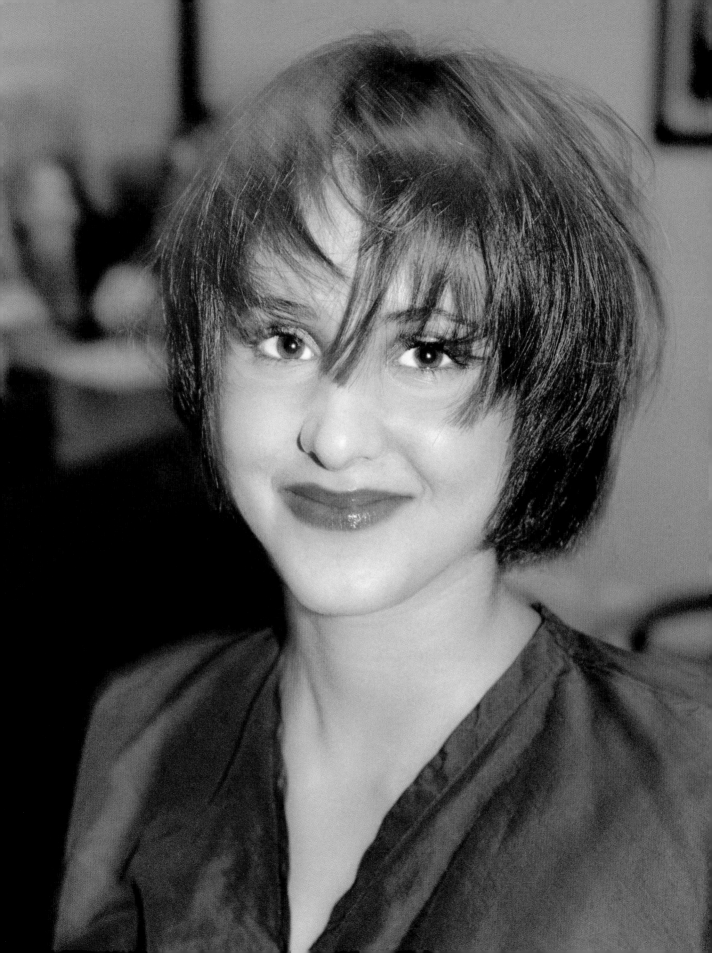

He happens to be a musician.

Deena, thirteen, is thinking she wants to reinvent herself as a rock star for this first date with the rock musician next door. She chose a funky, punk-angel style with popcorn hair rosettes and added pink hair extensions. (*Just twist individual little chunks of braided or unbraided hair in tiny circlets and secure with bobby pins. If you like, add hair extensions.*) A sheer, fur-trimmed blouse, black jeans, and Doc Martens boots finished her iconoclastic look.

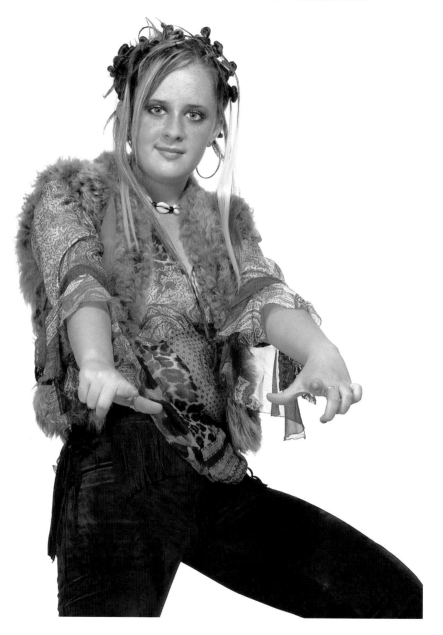

A Sweet Sixteen Sleep Over

My client **Melanie** told me about her sweet-sixteen party—a *Hair Today, Gone Tomorrow* sleep over. It was probably the best party she ever had, she said, because it became a try-this-look party—and there's nothing, she told me, that her friends would rather do.

We were inspired by Melanie's party, and so when I was invited to do some professional makeovers at another pajama party, I decided to have our ace photographer, Alex Cao, photograph the event.

First, Alex took pictures of each girl as she arrived in her street clothes, without makeup. Then, he took shots of the six girls as they did each other's nails and hair.

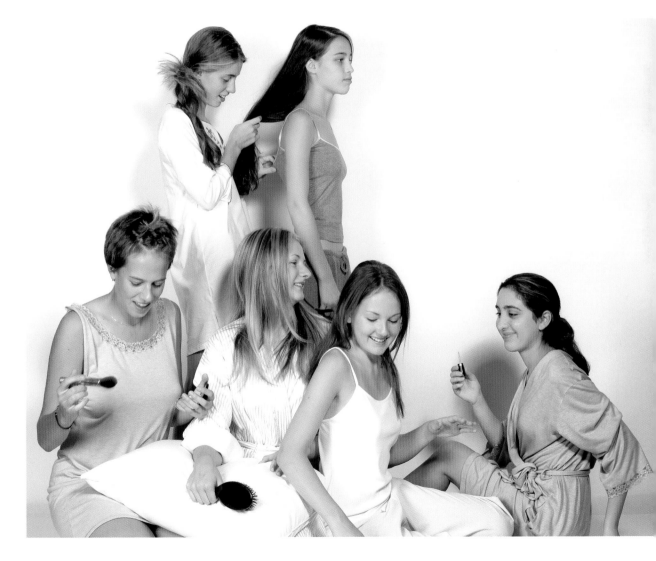

I'd made arrangements for them to stop off the week before at Saks Fifth Avenue (my home base), where they selected the outfits of their dreams in preparation for the *Cool Hair* pajama party shoot. The final photographs Alex took that evening were of all six teenagers as they looked playing dress up in their fancy duds and the transforming hairstyles I invented.

Getting together on a balmy spring evening, these fabulous teens had a blast as they played around with manicures, pedicures, makeup, and one or two pillow fights.

Eighteen-year-old **Alix** (below) goes to the American University in Paris, has two and a half boyfriends, and wants to be a child psychiatrist.

At right, Alix is wearing thin, corduroy, flowered pants and an ultrafeminine, off-the-shoulder Cynthia Steffe cotton lace eyelet blouse. The outfit calls for a wide leather belt and hoop earrings.

Her hair's romantic in a bun that's on one side. (So easy: Just twist a top layer of hair toward one side and make a doughnut shape by tucking the ends in through the doughnut. Secure with pins.)

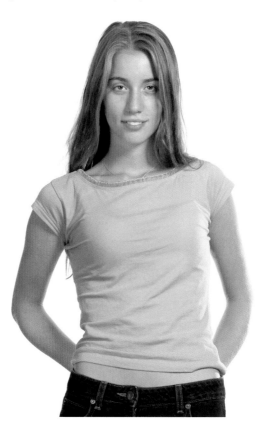

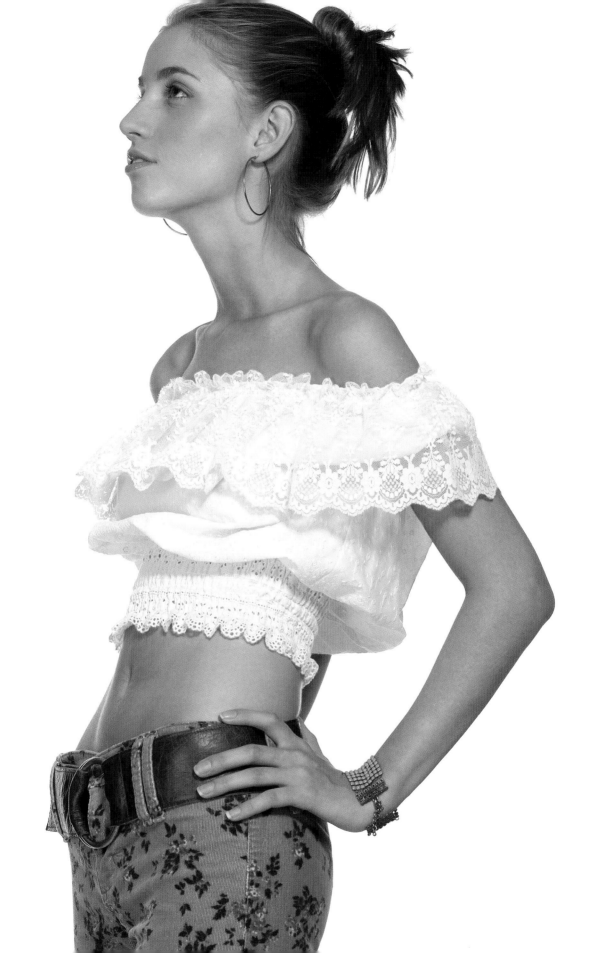

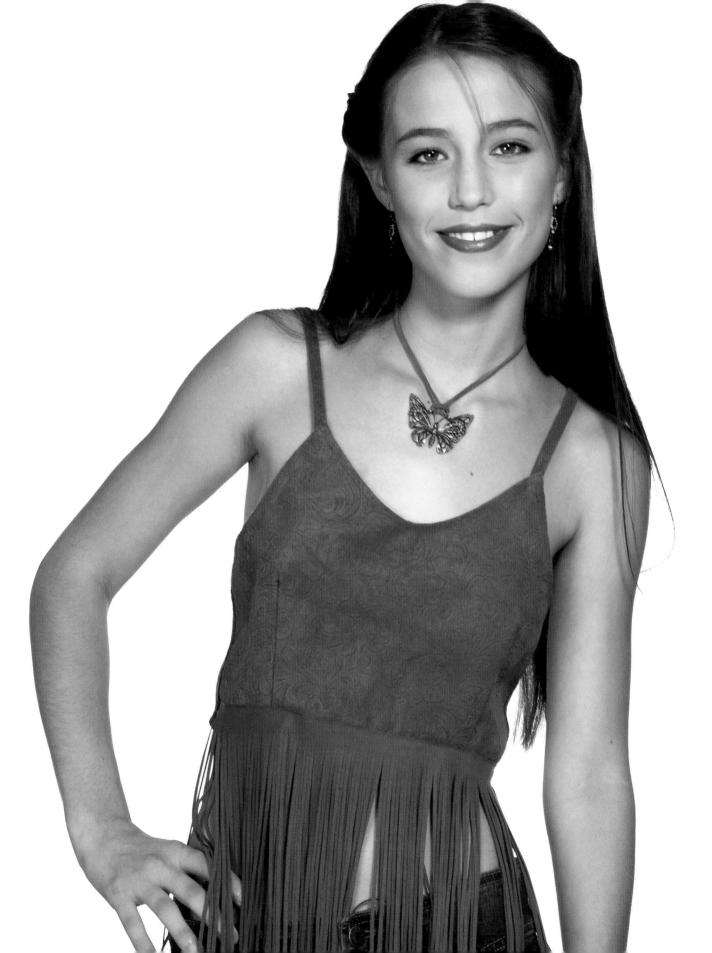

Victoria, thirteen, loves art, *La Scuola d'Italia,* where she goes to school, and how her long hair feels—she's been growing it since she was five.

Look at Victoria at left, who's now very "down on the range" in a cowboy-fringed embossed-suede camisole topping her low-rise jeans.

Boots, a suede rope at the hips, and a turquoise butterfly pendant are just the right accessory touches. I've isolated two small sections of her hair at each side, twisted them, and connected them at the back with a pretty barrette.

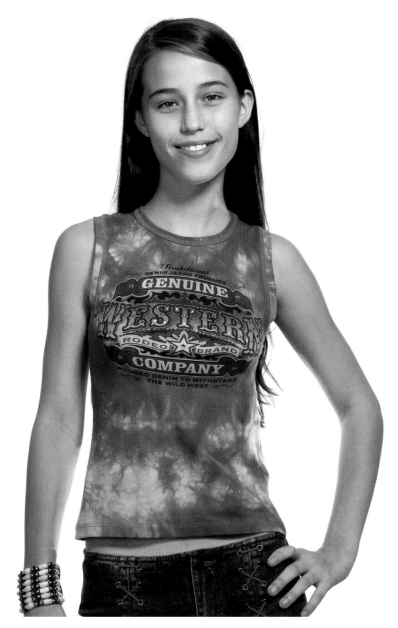

Sultry seventeen-year-old **Christina** is president of her school's model congress and is a political person with a double major in arts and poli sci. Her hero is her mom, who she thinks is so "passionate."

At right, after I blow-dry Christina's hair with a fat metal brush, this dark-haired beauty is now wearing a strawberry-cream tank over green, pink, and eggplant pants topped with a wide-wide leather belt and finished off with high-heeled sandals. Her huge hoop earrings are very stylish. Subtle golden lowlights (color, not bleach) in her hair lend radiance to her face.

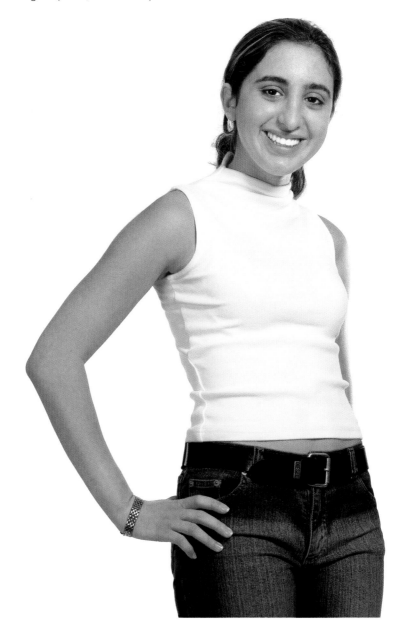

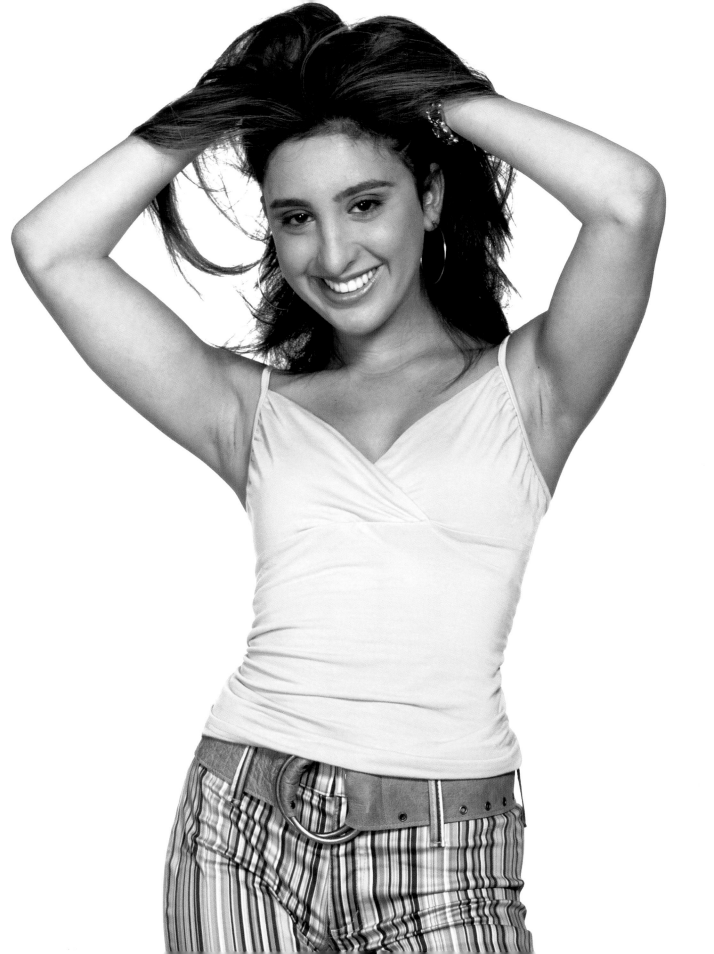

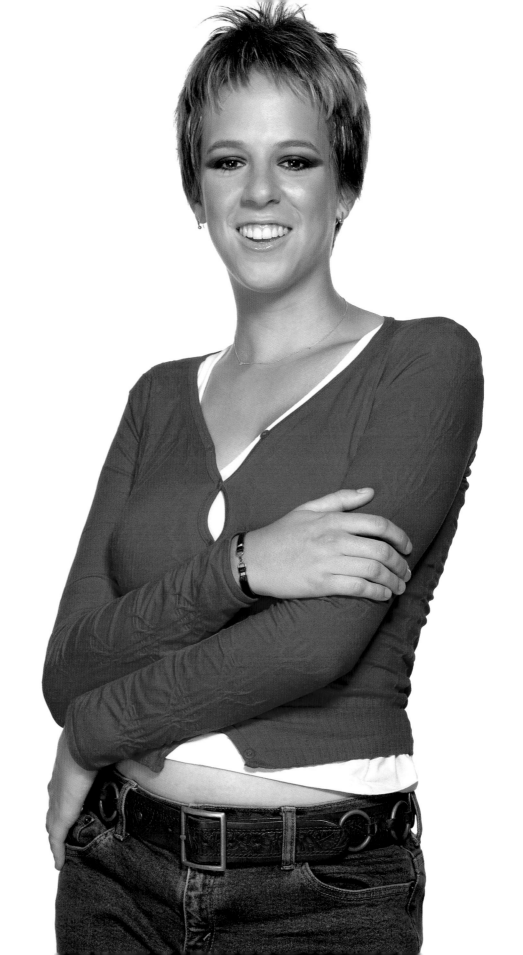

Helen, seventeen, is a lover of literature and studio art who adores exploring the big city by herself. She's an original—and she happily accepts her not-a-washboard body. The lower the hair maintenance, the higher her confidence level rises. She says she doesn't own a hairbrush.

At left, Helen has chosen to wear her own tomato-red sweater over a simple white T and jeans. I've also exaggerated her spiky, cute haircut by putting a little gel on the ends. Effect? Gamine combined with Voluptuous, which, on the pretty, interesting Helen, isn't a contradiction in terms.

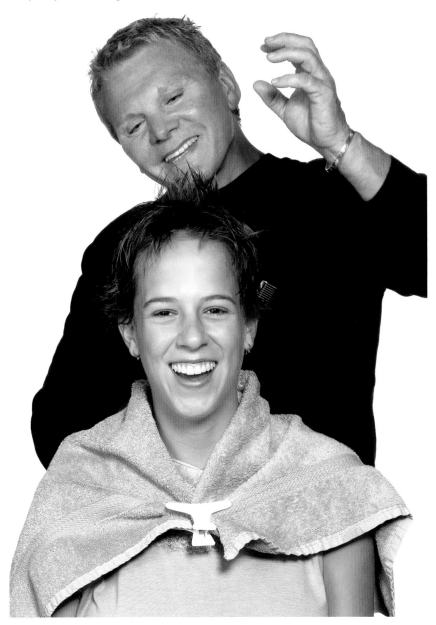

Erin, fifteen, is interested in fashion and singing. She's honest enough to say she cares a lot what people think. She feels most secure and confident when her hair looks good.

At right, here is Erin, transformed into a pre-Raphaelite beauty. After putting chunks of lighter highlights in her gorgeous tawny hair, I rolled it up in sections on a butane curling iron, held each section for ten seconds, then released the curling iron to get the *S* shapes (not curls), which I combed through with my ten fingers, no brush. She's wearing a marvelous black Moschino gown.

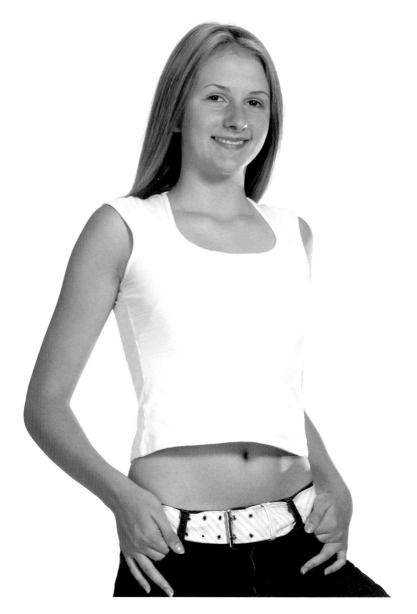

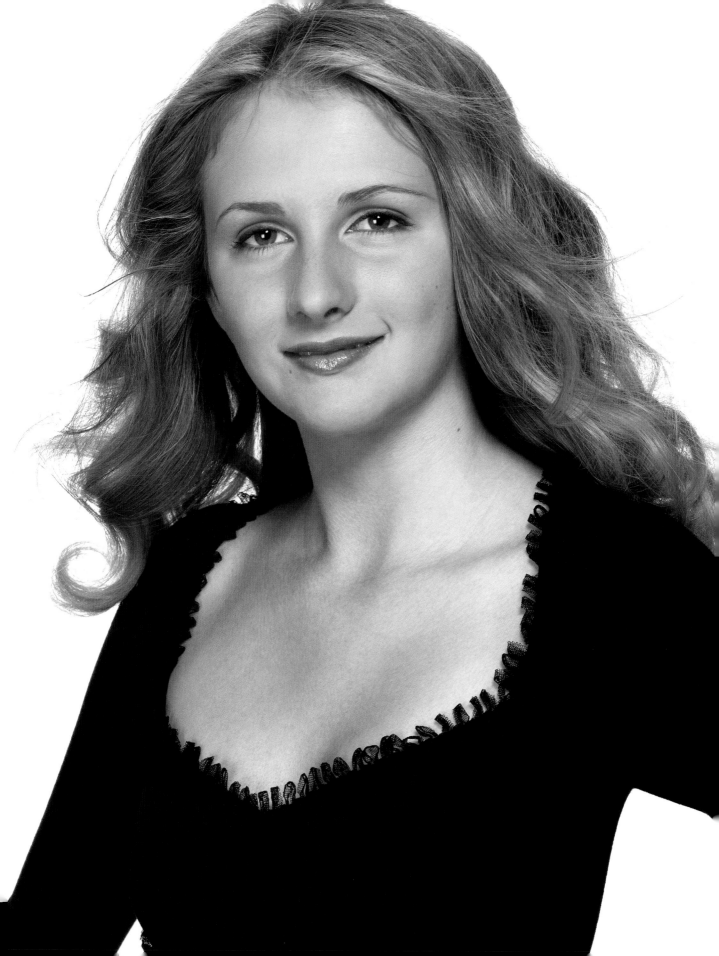

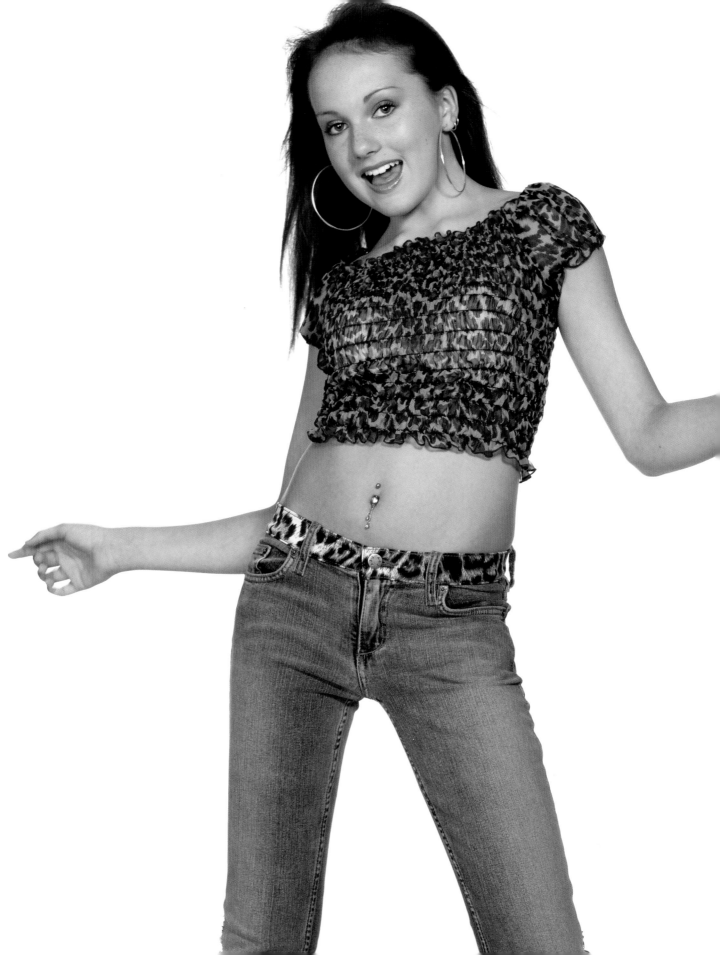

Then, there's thirteen-year-old, cute-as-a-button **Lauren**, who thinks she wants to be a model. That's this minute, anyway—next year, who knows? Maybe she'll be a brain surgeon.

At left, Lauren is now sporting a shirred leopard-print silk shirt ending just above her rhinestone-studded belly button. She's feeling, in her own words, "very grrrrr." Leopard-enhanced jeans finish that very animal look.

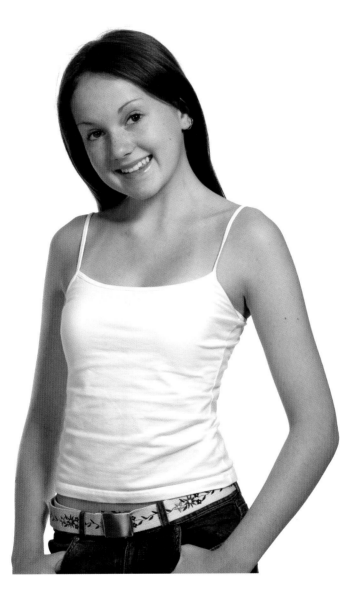

It was a great party. No sleeping at this pajama party. Just gossip, nail polish, and lots of blow-dryers.

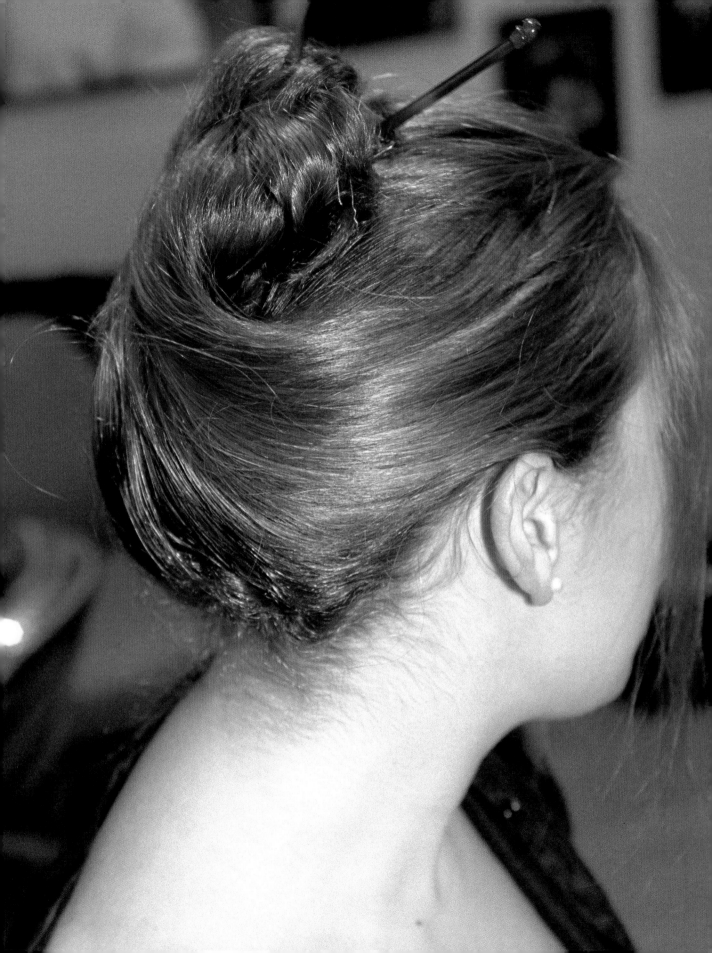

Hair grips can make a style, not to mention save a look, especially when the weather's so damp, your hair hasn't a chance. Ribbons, clips, and bows are marvelous for parties, but why wait for a party? You can buy many of these ornaments and wraps in any hair accessory section of your local drugstore or inexpensively in a beauty supply store. Further, if you are in the least creative, you can make your own.

So Get a (Pretty) Grip

Scrunchies: the cool version of yesterday's rubber bands, now encased in a tube of pretty fabric that squooshes up when you wrap it around your ponytail, bunches, braids, etc. Scrunchies come in a wide variety of fabrics, from velvet and elegant pleated silk to denim, chiffon, and cotton.

Bendies: long bendable wires wrapped in fabric that can be twisted around the hair. You can braid bendies into a ponytail, wrap one around a bun, or use them to finish off bunches or braids.

Headbands: indispensable to every length hair, and of course they're available in a huge variety of fabrics, materials, and widths. There's nothing like a headband to save a look when it's wilting.

Snap Wraps: These are Revlon products that are just wonderful for ponytails and bunches. They're brightly colored circlets with small combs attached inside. Make your ponytail and secure it with a covered elastic (plain rubber bands can pull out hair). Open the *Snap Wrap,* insert its tiny comb into the elastic, and you have a bright, ribbony band that controls even the wildest of tails.

Six-inch clips: The length of these barrette-clips makes them so useful in

Pretty Samantha with chopsticks.

securing chignons. They're colorful, and they gather, lift, secure, and dress up your hair.

Combs: Very vintage and, at the same time, very cool, combs are used to lift the hair off the face, allowing it to fall free but not in your eyes. Pretty combs also hold any upswept style with elegance.

Jeweled or sequined combs: These are tiny combs adorned with glitter, jewels, and shining color that add interest and life to your hair.

Barrettes: Choose the sleekest, simplest designs for everyday wear: topped with leather, grosgrain ribbon, velvet, or embossed metal. Fussy shapes are not elegant.

Hair tattoos: Every now and then, you come across a product that's just plain fun. If you ever see hair tattoos, grab them! These small and colorful appliqués come in the shapes of stars, moons, fish, turtles, and butterflies—you name it. When moistened, they can be applied to the hair—and even the forehead. They're so charming, they brighten up the mood of anyone who sees you and invite the inevitable question: "What's that and where did you get it?"

Make your own: Often, the best hair accessories are those you fashion yourself. Here are some ideas:

- Pretty fabrics and trimmings can be found in sewing and craft stores. Look for strips of sequins, colored beads, pearls, flowers, ribbons—and a glue gun to easily fasten your selection to headbands and combs.

- Beads can be threaded right onto strands of your hair (with the help of a pal) or onto a thin, bendable wire and used to wrap around a ponytail.

- Attach fabulous silk flowers onto simple hair clips and use them as ponytail, chignon, or braid adornments. Pretty artificial flowers and, better still, fresh blooms can be inserted on top of an upswept style or pinned onto any braided style.

- Hair sticks or pretty chopsticks can be used to hold a chignon in place or decorate an upswept style. Scarves add drama and femininity to any braid or ponytail. You can tie a pretty scarf in a floppy bow at the base of your ponytail or just knot it around the base and let the ends cascade down. Also, that same scarf can be used as a headband—a fifties look that's new again.

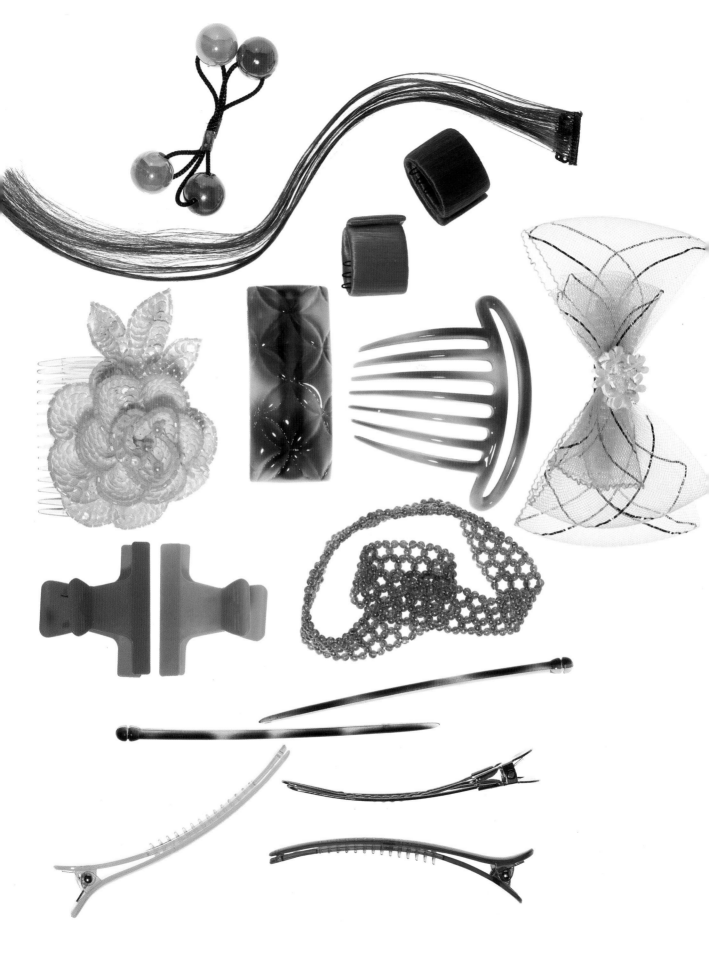

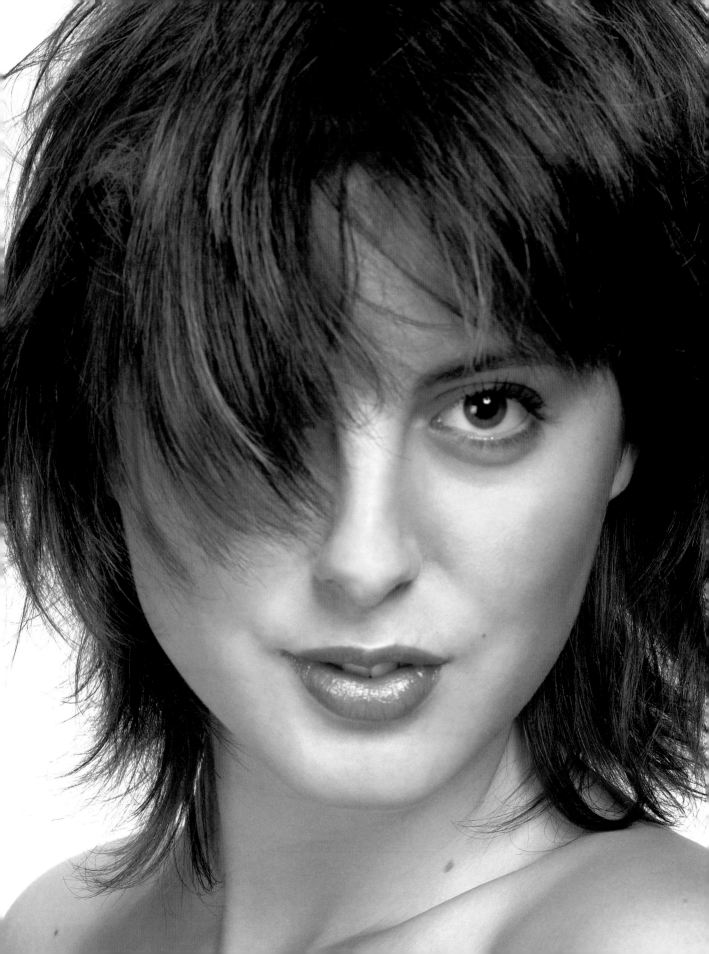

Radiant Skin | 9

I love hair. By now, you've figured that out. Nothing—I repeat, nothing—makes you prettier, sexier, or more self-confident than knowing your hair looks good. Coming in at a close second is knowing your face looks pretty. An amazing face comes from the character and energy of your personality, of course, but great skin and knockout makeup never hurt.

Superior skin always matters, and for that you need superior skin care. Take this quiz to see what you already know about skin.

Quiz

1. How much water do you drink every day?

   a. 2 to 3 glasses

   b. 6 glasses

   c. I drink mostly tea or coffee—and that is my fluid intake.

   d. I keep a large bottle of water in my backpack and am constantly sipping.

2. Answer true or false to the following statements:

   a. Never use soap when you wash your face and always use a toner and astringent.

   b. Even if your moisturizer or foundation has an SPF of 15 or over, you still need to regularly apply sunscreen when you're at the beach.

   c. It's best to wash your face at least four times a day.

   d. A good cream moisturizer puts needed moisture into the skin.

Eighteen-year-old Eva Amurri, Hollywood's newest star in *The Banger Sisters,* has just started college. She's got the gorgeous skin of your dreams . . . not to mention the sexy wild hair, the eyes, the personality, and the intelligence.

3. How much do you know about zits? Answer true or false to the following statements:

   a. Skin breakouts always come because you don't clean your face.

   b. Foods like greasy pizza, French fries, and chocolate are zit makers.

   c. Some makeup can cause zits; some makeup can help get rid of zits.

   d. Keeping your skin as dry as possible is the best zit preventer.

   e. A good dose of sun helps get rid of pimples—but make sure you're wearing a sunscreen with an SPF of at least 15.

   f. It's okay to pop zits, *if* you do it carefully.

Answers and Analysis

Take 10 points for each correct answer.

1. Statements *b* and *d* are correct. The skin must have a large intake of water to be soft and clear of blemishes, and applying moisturizers doesn't do it (the moisture must come from inside). Neither does coffee or tea. The caffeine they contain has negative effects (jumpiness, higher blood pressure) that outweigh the good from the liquid.

2. a. False. Dermatologists recommend mild, nonirritating soap for normal skin (Basis, Dove, Purpose). If your skin is oily, consider a cleanser that contains salicylic acid or mild benzoyl peroxide, but always check with your dermatologist to make sure it's right for you. Also, if you have oily skin, use a non- or low-alcohol astringent like witch hazel occasionally. Not everyone needs it: In fact, overuse of witch hazel may cause sebaceous glands to produce even more oil.

   b. True. Sunscreen should be applied to every exposed place—not just the face.

   c. False. Most of you need only to wash twice a day because too-frequent washing can strip skin of protective moisture. If your skin is superoily, wash three times or use a cleanser for oily skin.

   d. False. Moisturizers seal water into your skin, which is why you should apply them to a damp face.

3. *Take 5 points for each correct answer.*

   a. False. Breakouts can be caused by your genes, tension, or normal oil production—not only by lack of cleanliness.

   b. False. No scientific experiment has ever proven that certain foods cause zits—no matter what your mom says.

   c. True. If you have a zit problem, look for makeup that is noncomedogenic (it won't clog your pores). Certain cosmetic products contain salicylic acid that treats and prevents breakouts.

   d. False. Zits are pores that are clogged with oil from under the skin's surface. Keeping your skin dry on the outside doesn't stop those oil glands from producing pore-clogging oil, especially during adolescence.

   e. False. A good dose of sun does nothing good for your skin and may be very dangerous for it. In fact, it may make breakouts worse by thickening the skin, making it easier for pores to clog. Sunlight doesn't do even one helpful thing to fight acne or zits.

   f. False. Popping zits can irritate oil glands, produce swelling, and actually create new zits. It can scar your face. It's a nasty habit. But some of you will still do it, no matter what I say. See page 123.

Did you score from 60 to 80? You're very skin savvy and I'm proud of you. When you're sixty, I bet your skin will look thirty.

Did you score from 35 to 55? You do about as well as most teens when it comes to skin care smarts—and that means you could do better. After you finish reading the chapter, you'll be brilliant!

Did you score 30 or under? You're sabotaging your skin by carelessness, and you need to catch up to your more skin-sophisticated sisters.

The Skin You're In

There are lots of fascinating facts about skin. For starters, skin is the largest organ in the body and certainly the most visible. What's most interesting is that at one time or another, over 90 percent of all girls have acne—just a fancy word for pimples—so you're not alone if you have just sprung a zit.

No makeup in the world will look terrific if the skin beneath it is not at least pretty good. I'm about to tell you how to have better than pretty-good skin. My system will bring you *very* good skin.

The Vincent Skin Care System

Cleanliness is the basis of good skin. Because you're a teenager, you already know that you're subject to rising hormones that cause impacted oil glands and subsequent skin eruptions. Sometimes, bad skin is simply genetic. Sometimes, you've done yourself in with too many late nights, too much alcohol or cigarettes, or by being less than diligent about your cleansing habits. Your skin may change as you get older. If it's oily, it may dry out some. If you treat it and clean it as it exists right now, you can go a long way toward avoiding zits. Skin must be cleaned, moistened, and well nourished.

Everyone cleans her skin in different ways depending on her skin type. But everyone should moisten skin in the same way—by drinking lots of water and by using moisturizing products to seal in the water you pat on your face. Of course, we all should nourish our skin by eating good food.

Skin Types and Cleansing Tips

Oily Skin

If your nose is shiny when you wake up, you have oily skin. The good news is that your skin will look more supple and younger longer than the dry skin of your pals. Still, you have to cleanse deeply, although not too often, to avoid those breakouts. Strange as it seems, if you wash too often—especially if you use strong oil-stripping soaps—you'll only increase oil production and aggravate those zits. Try washing no more than twice daily with a mild, nonfoaming, detergent-free, fragrance-free cleanser. A no-detergent soap like Neutrogena can be used for normal to oily skin. Or try an oil-free gel cleanser containing a pore declogging ingredient like salicyclic acid or a pimple fighting solution like 1 to 3 percent glycolic acid. Your druggist can help you find products with these ingredients, but one I like is Neutrogena *Oil-Free Acne Wash*. Never use scented soap—only unscented. Fragrance can be a major skin irritant.

Dry Skin

Since you're a teenager, chances are your skin won't be all that dry, but if it's very sensitive and feels tight and irritated after you wash your face, you might indeed have a dryness problem. Please don't spend a fortune on ointments, placenta creams, cocoa butter, and whatever else you read will moisturize your skin. It won't. Cleanse daily with a nonastringent cleanser on a soft

Lindsay Anderson.

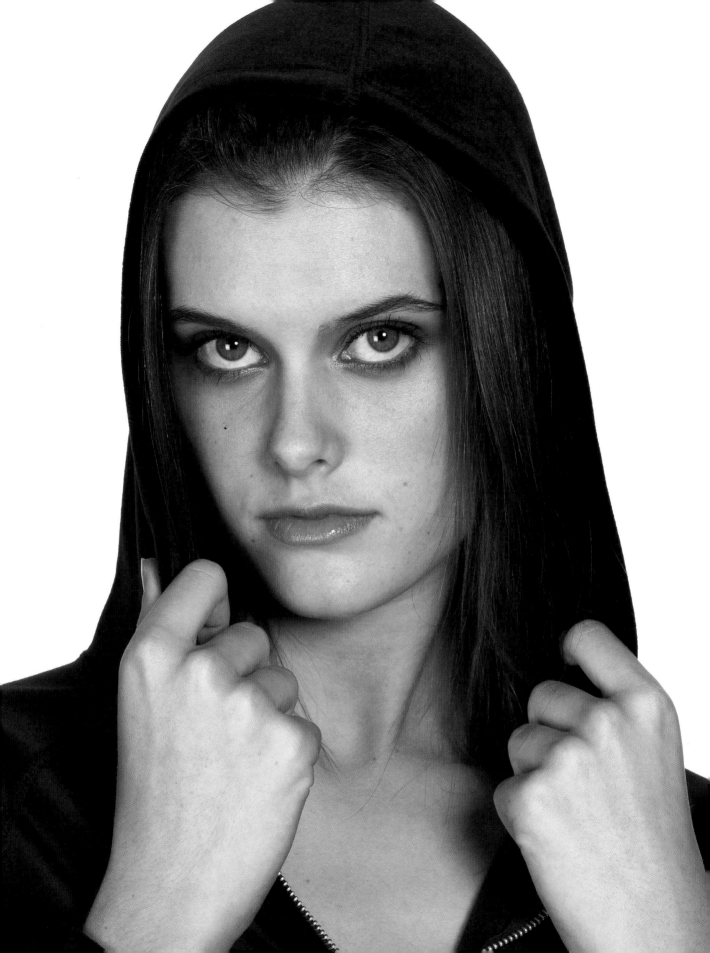

Tips for Oily Skin

Ever see a rock star with pimples? Not likely.

They have their ways, but check with a dermatologist to see if their ways should be your ways.

- Deep-pore cleansing strips: Use them no more than once a week to help get out the guck from areas that have caused trouble before, but never, never, never use a pore strip on areas that are already broken out. (Bioré, Jergens, and Neutrogena put out good strips.)

- Ask your druggist for a lotion containing antibacterial 2.5 percent benzoyl peroxide. Apply a thin layer to your skin at night to areas where you have a tendency to break out.

- For really oily skin, most rock stars and models in the know skip the moisturizing products altogether. If you must use a moisturizer, try an oil-free one. I like Elizabeth Arden's *Matte Moisture Lotion*. Remember: Moisturizers don't really provide moisture, they just seal it in. The best way to provide moisture to your skin is by drinking at least seven to eight glasses of water a day. When those rock stars dash offstage for a moment, they're grabbing a drink of water. Trust me.

- If you are breaking out around your chin a whole lot, your lifeline—the telephone—could be the villain. Bacteria just love to breed on that receiver! Wipe the phone with alcohol pads every day, and try not to touch the receiver to your chin when you talk.

- African American skin is naturally more oily and more prone to breakouts. It also has more pigment, which means it scars easily (and often permanently, so *never* fool with your zits). Ask your dermatologist about using a daily cleanser containing salicylic acid.

- I like Elizabeth Arden's *Oil-Control Refining Cleanser*; use it twice daily. Arden's *Zap It* blemish control reduces the inflammation from pimples and speeds healing, say many of my clients.

- Carry a pack of mildly astringent cleaning pads in your backpack. They cut down on oily face shine.

- The pimples on your chest or back should be treated just like those on your face. Clean often and apply an acne-control product nightly.

- Towels and washcloths should be fresh and clean for each use. Remember, bacteria is just as much a culprit as oil.

Tips for Dry Skin

- Use a humidifier at night or put a pan of water on the radiator.

- Use a treatment with alpha hydroxy acid every week or so to rid the skin of dead skin cells.

- Winterize your skin by remembering never to go out in the cold, sleet, or snow without a moisturizer with an SPF of at least 15. Elizabeth Arden's *Eight Hour Cream* soothes dry skin irritation and symptoms of windburn, sunburn, and chapping.

- Summer-proof your skin by using a sunblock with an SPF of 30 (I like Arden's *Triple Protection Oil-Free Sun Block*) and maybe even a light foundation.

- To keep pores clean and your face free of dry-skin flakes, use a mild scrub weekly before you moisturize. If you notice redness, stop using the scrub.

- If you *have* to use soap to feel clean, use a clear, transparent one like Pears or Neutrogena or a superfatted one like *Dove*.

- Elizabeth Arden puts out an incredibly lightweight revitalizer. It's a morning treatment, *Good Morning Skin Serum,* great after a grimy, grim, all-nighter study session. Drab and tired-looking skin perks up!

- Apply Vaseline or baby oil to slightly dampened skin to make it feel moister and softer in the morning.

- Drink at least eight glasses of water daily—especially essential if you have dry skin.

cloth. When you rinse your face in the morning, leave a thin layer of water on your skin, then seal it in with a product like Elizabeth Arden's *Ceramide Time Capsule Moisture Cream*.

Combination Skin

Approximately 70 percent of teens have combination skin, so you're in good company if this is your skin type. Combination skin is known for getting seriously confused. The T zone (forehead, nose, and chin) may be glistening with oil, while the rest of your face seems normal to dry and flaky. Cleansing it can be tricky. Instead of soap, use a mild, soap-free cleanser, such as Origins'

Result: The healthy skin gets red and irritated. Follow directions when using medicated products.

6. *Getting hair spray on your face.* As you spray your hair, protect your face. Many hair sprays, leave-in conditioners, and spray hair gels have oils and other ingredients that can clog skin pores. When spraying your hair, first cover your face with a paper towel or shield your face with your hand. Wash your face immediately if any hair product accidentally gets on your skin.

How to Camouflage Not-So-Bad Zits

Not every zit is a monster. Not-so-bad pimples can be "vanished" with a little ingenuity. I suggest a stick foundation (like those made by Max Factor or Bobbi Brown) for a just-starting culprit. Buy it in a shade that matches your skin color.

1. Dab it on the pimple with a small brush and also on the skin around the pimple. Then blend the dots and pat lightly with translucent powder. If the zit is a little larger, use a concealer instead of stick foundation. Some concealer comes only in light shades—this can make the zit stand out, much like your bottom in white jeans. Blot the too-light concealer twice after applying, which usually takes care of this problem. Dot some foundation on top to blend.

2. If your pimple is on its way out, you'll probably have flaky skin surrounding it. Smooth on some waxy, clear lip balm to help the foundation and powder stick to the area.

3. Before you go to sleep, put ice in a washcloth and gently rub it over the pimple to reduce the inflammation. Then, mix a half teaspoon of dry yeast (buy in a health food store) with a few drops of water and apply the paste to the pimple. In the morning, rinse. It works—but I can't tell you why.

But Big, Bad Zits Do Happen

Sometimes, no matter what you do, serious zits happen. When they happen just before a big event, you're not going to listen to anyone who tells you not to squeeze, peel, or pop them. I know that.

Even though it's much better not to, here are some guerilla tactics for when you just *have* to.

Zit Busters

If there's no visible pus, forget it. All the popping/squeezing/pushing in the world will only bring you more grief in the form of scars. When you squeeze pimples that are not ready to burst, although some stuff will come out, you're also forcing that zit to rupture backward into the tissue—a sure precursor to serious acne and scarring—and maybe even worse—infection.

If some pus *is* visible, apply a hot washcloth to the area for ten minutes, remove, let skin cool for ten minutes, and repeat for two hours. This brings white blood cells to the area and speeds healing. The warmth may bring the pimple to a head. (Don't use a pin—even a sterilized pin—or your nails to squeeze. It won't work and it will make the zit even more visible.)

If this doesn't work, that pimple's going nowhere. Give up and use a concealer (see page 122).

If the pus is gone but now you've got a big red blotch where the zit used to be, apply witch hazel, then ice to reduce the swelling and redness. Then apply concealer.

If you have time, and you're seriously desperate, ask your dermatologist if there's anything that can be done to make the offender go away—like a cortisone shot. If the answer is no, be a big girl. Your date has had such a zit himself, I promise you. It will not come as a shock to him. He'll understand.

If you have a chest breakout, the culprit is perspiration in that area. Try to wear cotton bras and T-shirts—at least for a while. They absorb the perspiration so it doesn't sit on your chest, doing damage. Wash the whole area twice daily. Apply a facial mask to the chest area weekly to clean out the pores.

News flash: If you have inflammatory acne (the kind that looks like angry red bumps), the FDA has just approved a brand-new and effective light-based therapy that causes the bacteria in acne to self-destruct. It's called *Clear-Light*. This painless therapy, an alternative to topical creams and antibiotics, is a high-intensity lamp directed at the acne. Check with your dermatologist.

Pimples Love Anxiety

If you've gotten the impression that good skin takes work, you're right. There are always those fortunate teenagers who have that clear-faced radi-

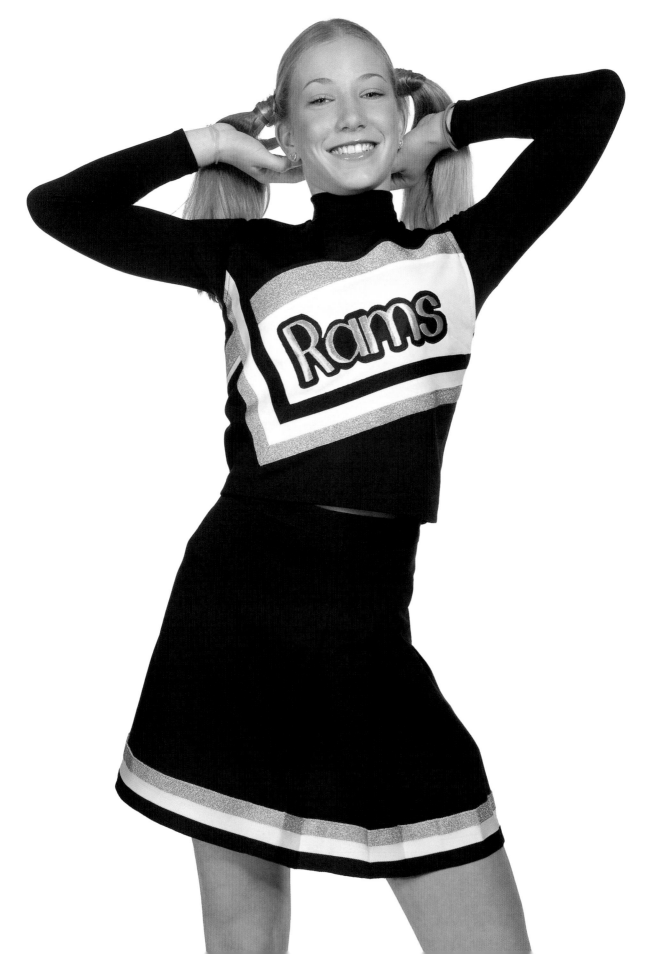

ance without even thinking about it—let alone cleansing properly—but for most of you, developing or maintaining good skin requires time and effort. What you do now lays the foundation for the way your skin will glow the rest of your life.

If you are doing everything right and your skin is still giving you problems: Don't stress out about it. This may be easier said than done. It can be emotionally traumatic to have flare-ups of acne, and it takes a very strong girl not to be anxiety ridden when you have to live with pimples and blotches. Remember that anxiety's power to worsen skin conditions has been well documented in clinical studies, so the cooler you can stay emotionally, the clearer your skin will be.

While you're waiting for your skin to clear up, try not to pick or pop pimples, or peel your face. The good news is this: It *will* clear up. The skin you're in as a teenager can only get better as you head into your late teens and early twenties.

Jenn has naturally radiant skin.

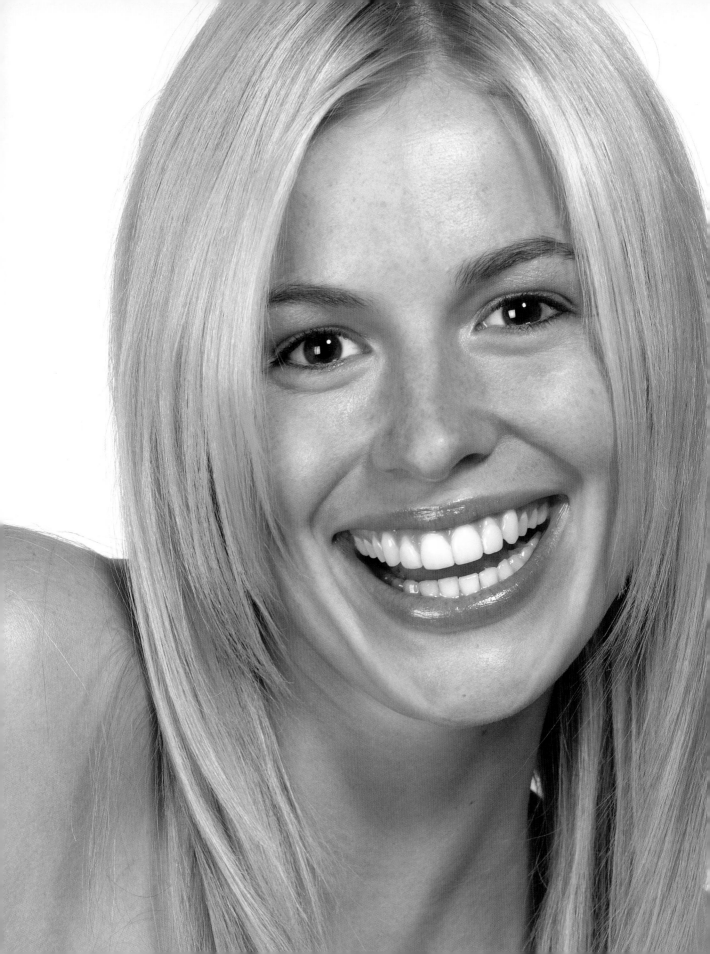

Amazing Face | 10

Cleopatra did it. Also Nefertiti and Ophelia, although it was against Hamlet's wishes. The ancient Egyptians wouldn't be caught embalmed without their pots of black kohl. Christina Aguilera, Mandy Moore, and Kate Hudson do it. Kelly Osbourne definitely does it. Even the fresh-faced Olsen twins—otherwise known as Mary-Kate and Ashley—do it.

Do what? Paint their faces, that's what, otherwise known as use makeup. Even in the most prudish times, girls have found ways to moisten and color their faces with natural lubricants and berries. Women have been wearing makeup for centuries for one reason: It makes them look pretty. Take the most natural-faced movie star and I guarantee I could scrape off about two pounds of carefully applied makeup from her amazing face. It just *looks* as if she's makeup free.

We're talking about putting on *your* best face, your most amazing face. It is possible to have an amazing face. Even if you've never before thought of yourself as beautiful, the extraordinary new products available, and the freedom with which most teens experiment with makeup, give you endless opportunities to become beautiful, cute, sexy, interesting—whatever part of *amazing* you choose. The colors; the glimmer; the dazzle; the shimmer; the sultry, smoky shades; the bright berry looks; the subtle, natural glows are all out there, waiting for you to dip in. What are you waiting for?

First, what's your makeup signature, and what can I tell by your choices?

QUIZ: What's Your Makeup Signature?

1. What lip gloss flavor is most you?

    a. Cool peppermint

Eighteen-year-old Pam Brown has it all—the face, the hair, the style, and the smile. Also, she's a writer. An amazing teen.

b. Spicy cinammon

c. Sensual passion fruit

d. Flavorless

e. Sparkling wine

2. What lipstick shade best defines you?

a. The Frost is On the Rose

b. Tangy Terra Cotta

c. Jungle Red Alert

d. Neutral Lip Balm

e. Tarty Tangerine

3. What's your usual makeup routine?

a. I rarely wear makeup.

b. I love to experiment and take my time; if you have a fun style or color to try, bring it here!

c. Dramatic eyes, deep lipstick shades, very little cheek color

d. A drop of lip gloss, a little eyeliner—and I'm done!

e. Depends on my mood—and my moods change daily. I usually like an edge with makeup, something to mark my individuality (lid glitter?).

4. How many makeup products do you usually carry around?

a. None

b. 1 to 3

c. 4 to 5

d. 6 to 9

e. More, on occasion

5. Who's your beauty icon?

a. Kelly Osbourne—she's radical cool

b. Halle Berry—she has the most natural glow

c. Nicole Kidman—a feminine princess

d. Janet Jackson—careful and controlled but heavyish makeup

6. What do you know about mascara? Answer true or false:

a. It's fine to use hair dye on eyebrows and eyelashes: After all, they're hair too.

b. If your mascara gets dried up, spit on the wand, then redip it in the container.

c. Blue (or other colored mascara) is crude and ugly.

Answers and Analysis

1 to 3. If you answered mostly *a*'s or *d*'s, you're somewhat uninterested in makeup. It may be because you value an almost completely natural look—and that's fine, and pretty, if it's what you think looks terrific. But maybe you're insecure and fearful of experimenting. If this is so, loosen up, chill out, and take some chances! Wearing pretty color on your face is what young women have been doing through the centuries because it's fun and makes them feel good. Whatever you decide, if it's really you deciding, it's the right choice! If it's self-consciousness talking, though, take some time to risk exploring the world of color.

If you answered mostly *b*'s, you're a happening teenager. Sounds as if you have high self-esteem.

If you answered mostly *c*'s, you're a sultry child with a "look" and an interesting attitude. I bet your hair color isn't what you were born with—am I right?

If you answered mostly *e*'s, you're an iconoclast—a vivacious individual who pretty much makes her own decisions in life.

4. An *a* answer makes me worry a little about you. What happens if there's an emergency makeup problem? Don't you care? *Care!* A *b* or *c* answer seems about right. You're prepared but not neurotic. A *d* answer is excessive; weed a few out. An *e* answer is silly. Why would you ever have to carry more than nine makeup products unless you're going to the *American Idol* tryouts?

5. I have no comment (except for one tiny thing) about these answers—you know whose look you like. But if you chose Kelly Osbourne, are you *sure*?

6. a. False. You could go blind!

b. False. That's the route to a major infection.

c. False. It can be witty, if the situation is right. I don't advise blue mascara for a job interview.

The Vincent Makeup

Before We Begin

My philosophy of makeup for teens (or post-teens or even their mothers) is *subtle, gentle, natural*. That's the most beautiful way to go.

Having said that, I also believe there are a few times when you want to look different, take a chance, go heavy-duty, double trouble on almost everything I'm going to talk about. When you're feeling funky; when you're experimenting

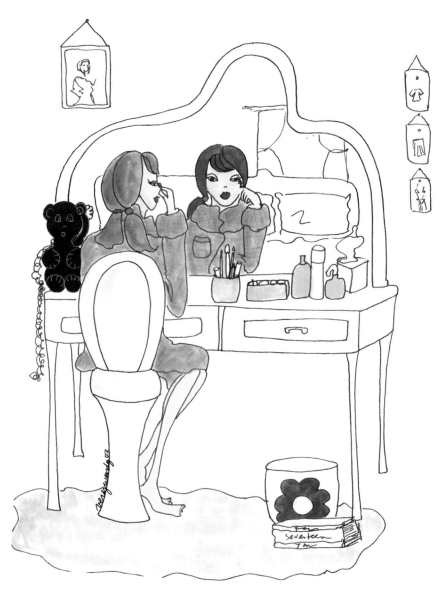

with friends; when you're going to a party where everyone is sure to rock; or when you're simply home alone playing with berry-red lips, smoky-gray raccoon eyes, or faux beauty marks, have fun.

Remember this: When it comes to makeup, the fast and steady rules are meant to be broken by girls who take chances and try out their own versions of *beautiful*.

For my makeup tips for the *most amazing face in town,* read on (but feel free to break any of my rules).

What You Need

You do not need nineteen lipsticks or thirty-two eye shadows. Simplify your life. Empty out your makeup bag. If you haven't worn a product in the last three months, lose it—you'll never use it. Start fresh. You should have:

- **4 lipsticks**—If you wear lipstick, one earthy brown-based shade, one true red, one soft pink, one peach. Many of my teen clients use only gloss.

- **4 lip glosses**—clear, ruby, pink, bronze. I like the gooey ones best—those that come in pots or wands are better than sticks or balms. These glosses are the mainstay of the teen makeup, usually used by themselves for the most natural look. If you go with lipstick, glosses on top can subtly change the shade as well as give a seductive glimmer.

- **2 foundations**—one cream foundation (like Max Factor's *Pan-Stick*) if you need more coverage for a blemish, and one water-based liquid type for daily wear. All foundation should always be in a shade that's a tad lighter than your natural skin color. Apply it with a damp sponge or your fingers, whichever works best for you. You can experiment with three to four water-based foundations and mix and match them until you get your exact color and then pour your combination, personally designed foundation into a fresh new plastic bottle that has a tight-fitting cover.

- **1 powder blusher**—in a soft rosy-pink shade

- **1 liquid concealer**—in a shade that's similar to your foundation

- **1 container loose powder**—if you use powder—and one translucent pressed-powder compact to carry

- **1 mascara**—black if your hair is very dark, brown if you have lighter hair. For disco nights try colored mascara—aquamarine or even white.

- **4 eye shadows**—experiment to see which colors are good for your eyes. I like toasty browns, soft greens, smoky grays, and golds. You can alternate between cream or powder shadows, even combining them for different looks, if you like.

I have not included lip-lining pencils. They were once very popular, but I don't use them. Even when blended in, they often give a coloring-book effect. Teens certainly shouldn't have lined lips.

Makeup Tools

You also need a few tools. I suggest:

- **Q-Tips** to erase mistakes, to apply concealer, to smudge eyeliner, for everything!

- **3 fat, fluffy, sable brushes**—one for powder, a smaller one for blusher, one for contour. It's important they be very clean. You can put them in the top level of the dishwasher, but remove them before the dry cycle.

- a small, supple, lip-color brush

- an eyelash curler

- a tweezer

- **makeup sponges**—natural, if possible

Preparing the Canvas

1. *Clean up your act!* First, cleanse your face. Then apply a very light layer of moisturizer (unless your skin is really oily) so the foundation will glide on more smoothly.

2. *Hide what needs to be hidden.* With your fingers, a Q-Tip, or a small sponge, dot and smooth concealer in a shade that matches your skin—or a tad darker, never lighter, wherever there's a blemish. I love a product called *Flawless Finish Concealer* from Elizabeth Arden. Dot it

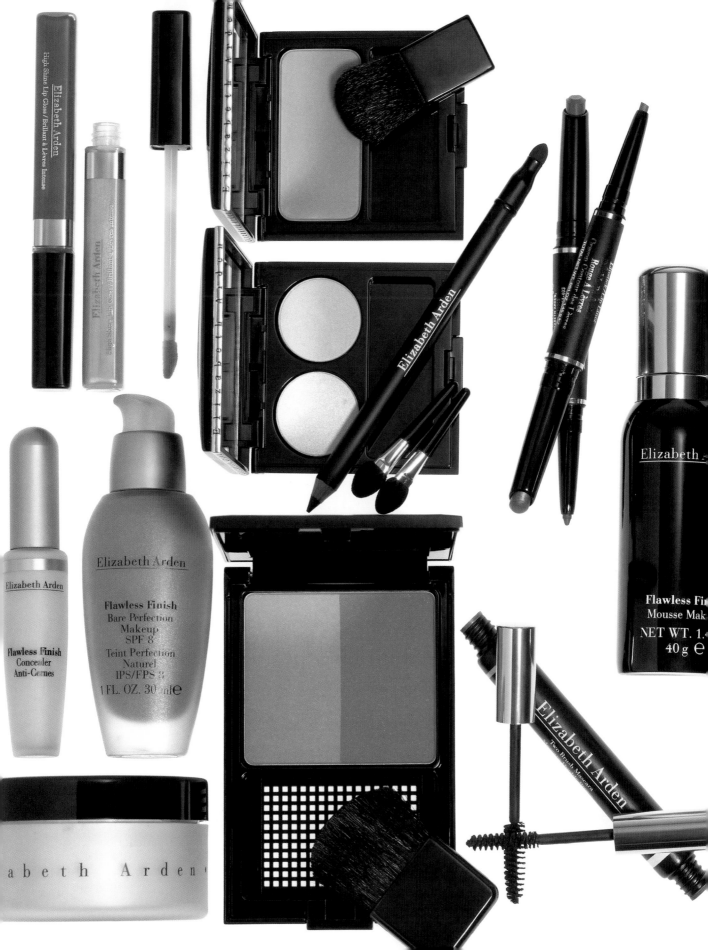

under eyes, on pimples, on burst blood vessels around the nose, on veins on the eyelids—you know what needs to be hidden. Blend, blend, and blend again. Visible spots of concealer look worse than blemishes—too-light concealer makes those zits glow. For really bad eruptions, try a medical concealer. (Covermark puts out a good one.) To keep your concealer from fading, dust it with translucent loose powder (this is one of the few times you'll use that loose powder).

3. *Paint the canvas*. Now the foundation. Apply some foundation. I often use Elizabeth Arden's *Flawless Finish Mousse Makeup* because it is so light and natural—like a real chocolate mousse. Spray or dab some on a dampened sponge and paint your face. Paint everywhere—your lips, neck, forehead, eyelids. The idea is to get an evenly painted canvas—not one that's blotchy or spotty. Check your face in natural light, if possible. Dot on a drop more concealer in the places you need it. Blend it into the foundation. Blend yet again, especially where the jawline meets the neck.

4. *Color!* Powder blusher on the cheeks gives you radiance—and brush a bit on your chin and forehead also. Clinique's *Gel Blush* is also very natural looking. Bronzer powder gives you a sun-kissed look, and that alone makes broken-out skin look better. Blend with a damp sponge.

5. *Powder!* With a fat fluff of a brush, apply a thin layer of matte translucent powder (either pressed or loose) to set everything, and blend yet again. Baby powder works if you run out of translucent powder. On especially oily areas like your nose, use blotting sheets before you apply powder. Many teens today go without powder, but I like a light powdering because it makes the makeup last.

6. *Tone*. Finally, if you think your hand was a little heavy with the makeup, a dampened sponge will tone it all down.

The Eyes

1. Curl your lashes *carefully* with a lash curler (never pull the lash curler away until it's open). With your finger (for cream shadow) or a small brush (for a powder shadow), apply color to your upper lids from the lash line to the crease and a teeny bit beyond. Don't try to match your eye color—blue shadow and blue liner don't do a thing for blue eyes.

For green eyes, try deep plum; for brown or black eyes, try moss green or charcoal; for blue or gray eyes, try coppery brown. Blend. For a special effect, a drop of shimmer to highlight the eye from brow to lash is always fun—and if you're feeling especially playful, a dab of that shimmer on the cheekbones and the center of the bottom lip is great. Stila's *Eye Glaze* comes in a handy pen with a soft tip that dispenses a pearly cream shadow.

2. Now, the eyeliner. Here's my special trick: Dip a soft, pointed brush into water, then into a charcoal or brown powder eye shadow; paint on the lash line for a natural, soft effect. Or use a pencil eyeliner, like Elizabeth Arden's *Powder Pencil,* which has a lovely smudger on one end. Draw a soft line right along—and even on—the lash line, starting about a third of the way from the inner corner of the eye. There should never be a space between your natural eyelash line and the painted one. No Cleopatra eyes please—don't let the liner wing out beyond the eyes. Gently smudge with a Q-Tip or sponge-tip smudger. To finish, I sometimes like to apply a bit of powder eye shadow on a Q-Tip and run it over the drawn line to blend and soften the effect.

3. Darken your lashes with a single coat of mascara in brown for fair skin, black for darker complexions, and colored for disco. Wedge the mascara wand into the roots of the lashes and shimmy it through to the tips. If any clumps remain, sweep them away with a tiny eyelash comb or an old mascara wand you've cleaned off. I love Shu Uemura's mascara, which lasts forever on your lashes, as well as Anna Sui's clear mascara with the silver glitter—just plain fun.

Those Lips

I strongly prefer simply a touch of clear or softly colored lip gloss for those luscious teenage lips. Elizabeth Arden's *High Shine Lip Gloss* is perfect, as is Urban Decay's *Lip Gunk.*

If you feel you must wear lipstick:

1. Apply a thin layer of foundation and then just a pat of translucent powder over your lips.

2. Apply the color. It's easiest to use the lipstick tube, but you can use a lip brush if you prefer.

3. Carefully blend and blot.

4. Take your lip brush (or your finger) and dip it into a pot of gloss. Then, delicately, dot onto your bottom lip. If you glop the gloss thickly all over your mouth, your mouth will look like an ice-skating rink.

And that's the Vincent makeup.

The Lighter Touch

I've given you the basics of a very full makeup, wonderful especially for evening occasions. Many teenagers prefer to go a lot lighter for every day, and I agree that it's far better to let your own natural beauty shine through than be overpowered by color in the daylight hours. If you must use foundation to even out the color on a skin that may be blotchy and broken out, use just the barest covering so your natural coloring is visible. If you must use eyeliner, use pencil and not liquid, and gently smudge the line with a Q-Tip or smudger so the line looks soft. Daytime mascara should be a subtle darkening of your natural lashes—no fringes please. The lightest of lipsticks or, better yet, mere gloss should be on your mouth, making it luscious and kissable.

I admire your look! I admire your confidence!

Road Test a Cosmetic

How many raindrops in a thunderstorm? That's the number of cosmetic choices you have to try before you adopt them for your very own. You can road test certain products right in the department stores. For example, you can safely test a foundation or blusher by asking the salesperson for a clean sponge to apply the product, but do not use the tester lipstick on your mouth—think how many maybe-not-so-clean mouths it's been on! Use your judgment.

Product Rip-offs, Hoaxes, and—Whoaaaa, It's-a-Miracle—Creams

You really have to use your head when you're dealing with your face. The cosmetics market is probably the steadiest, richest, fastest-growing industry in all the world; that's because every girl and woman wants to look pretty. The

Samantha's makeup is polished but natural.

bad news is that in many ways, it may also be the scamiest market. If you're buying makeup and skin care products, you've always got to read between the lines; and if something sounds too good to be true, it probably is. Huge advertising budgets and clever advertisements don't necessarily make a product terrific—just expensive. The good news is that you don't have to spend a fortune to find the freshest, most flattering products; often, the least expensive lipstick is the coolest.

Experiment, experiment, experiment, but in the meantime, here are some common hoaxes and product rip-offs to watch out for:

Just Say No If:

- any makeup or skin care product insists that you must buy the whole line, the whole system, the whole shebang or else be smothered in pimples. Even when reputable manufacturers say it makes *scientific* sense to buy all your skin care and cosmetic needs from one company, it doesn't.

- any company says that its bizarre and exotic extracts will work wonders on you. Stay away from the company's chicken placenta/seaweed/quail egg/turtle and mink oil/honeybee extract and horse sperm creams at a zillion dollars a jar.

- soaps promise miracles. Moisturizing soaps don't contain moisture (which is simply water), but oil that gets washed down the drain with the first rinse. Medicated soaps are generally useless because that medication also gets washed away with the first rinse. Antibacterial soaps can actually do damage because they've been known to kill the skin's natural helpful bacteria. Perfumed soaps and shampoos are usually detergent products that can irritate skin and scalp better than anything else I know. Just say no if they try to soft-soap you.

- any product says it does too many things. How can a product be a cleanser (which means it has to open pores) and also be an astringent (which means it has to close those pores) at the same time? Think before you plunk down hard-earned cash—and just say no if the promises or the hype you hear or read make you squirm. Trust your judgment.

Makeup Tips

- Although there are tons of lip glosses and lip moisturizers out there, I know a dozen famous young women who swear by an application of honey over their lips and even over their lipstick. Tastes terrific. Other young women squeeze the contents of a vitamin E capsule on a finger and apply it to their lips as gloss: This also works as a healing agent for chapped lips.

- Unruly eyebrows? Lightly spritz an old toothbrush with hair spray, then brush brows into shape. Never spray directly onto your brows. A dab of chapstick brushed up with a toothbrush also works.

- Mix a couple of drops of moisturizer with a couple of drops of red-eye reliever and dot onto blemish area before applying concealer (it will stick better). Apply a drop of concealer and over that, foundation, then dot on more concealer. Pat translucent powder over pimple. What pimple?

- Need to clip your hair back while you apply makeup? Insert a facial tissue folded in half under each hair clip so you don't end up with dented hair.

- Want something a little extra on your face for disco night? Try face jewelry as beauty marks. Find little fake jewels (a ruby heart, a blue star, a green triangle) and paste them on with surgical glue.

- An ice cube massaged on red, puffy, after-a-cry eyes makes the puffiness disappear.

- If you're African American try a reddish-coral, *never orange,* blusher or gray, turquoise, or navy blue on your eyelids. Your skin has reddish and blue tints. Those makeup colors will look gorgeous on you.

- Want lush-looking lashes? Line the upper lash line with black or brown pencil; then wiggle the tip of the pencil between the lashes, darkening the skin between and making the lashes look thick.

- Teeth may not be makeup but they have everything to do with your face and *presentation*. Brush after every meal. A battery-powered electric toothbrush is terrific. Do you have braces? The cutest girls do. Just think how gorgeous your teeth are going to be when they're straight. And, when the braces do come off, if you're not happy with the whiteness level of your teeth, there are many new treatments available. Discuss it with your dentist. What you *can* do something about while you're waiting for those braces to come off is bad breath—common in teens. Brush, floss, and use mouthwash at least three times a day. Try a new product called Wrigley's *Eclipse* flash strips, a paper-like strip that instantly melts in your mouth and gives you cinnamon/spearmint /whatever breath. If there's still a halitosis problem, your dentist will have some ideas.

- it's smelly or oily. Products that are supposed to be for teen skin ought to be for teen skin—and that means fragrance free and, for oily skin, oil free. Read the ingredient label to be a savvy consumer.

Just Say Yes If:

- the makeup artist in the department store wants to give you a free makeup, even if she's pushing a particular brand. You might learn a lot, and the worst thing that can happen is that you have to wash your face to remove the finished product if you hate the result. So what if she's selling certain products? You don't have to buy a thing, and it's one of the few true freebies the cosmetics companies give away in order to make friends and *maybe* some sales.

Break These Rules

- *Your lipstick and nails should match your outfit.* Rule from the last century. It's much more interesting to contrast colors—coral lips and ruby nails rule.

- *The color lady says fair-complexioned blond girls should wear earthy makeup tones, and darker girls should stick to pink and rosy tones.* If you believe that, you'll buy this bridge I have to sell. Anyone can wear any color she likes if she finds the shade that lends her radiance.

- *Dab on some powder for a shiny nose.* First, remove the oil with an oil-blotting paper—then dab on the powder.

- *Eyeliner inside the eye rim makes your eyes look huge.* No, it doesn't. It only makes your eyes tear and eyeliner smudge.

- *Superlong claw nails are in.* Wrong, they're out.

About Your Emergency Backpack Stuffer

Every girl should have a small, flat container in her backpack stuffed with the absolute core necessities. We're not talking major makeover supplies here, just the quick touch-up ingredients. You need:

- your favorite lipstick (in a pinch, it doubles as a blusher) and lip gloss

- a pressed-powder/foundation combo in one tiny mirrored compact

- tissues, baby wipes, and one or two Q-Tips

- a tiny brush and comb for an instant back-combed hair lift

- breath mints

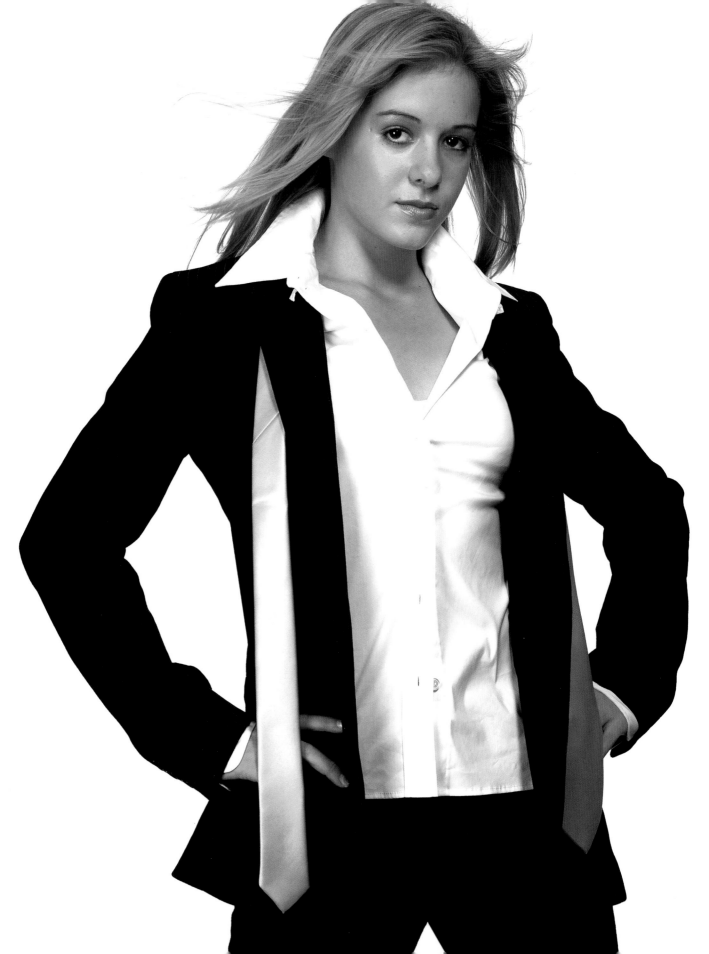

Dear Vincent | 11

Every day, I get asked questions by my teenage clients, and often they're the same questions. Usually they have to do with beauty, but sometimes they're more personal. I cherish all those young friends who trust me enough to listen to my thoughts on their problems. Here are some frequently asked questions:

You ask: In the winter, I have terrible, horrible, very bad, no good, flat, hat hair. How do I deal with hat hair?

Vincent:

- With a butterfly clip or barrette, clip the front section of your hair on top of your head before putting on the hat. When you're ready, remove both the hat and the clip and you'll be amazed at how much volume and lift remains.

- Choose a hat that "breathes"—lets air flow through. Cotton baseball caps are great for the beach and open cars. Cool shades are terrific with any hat, by the way.

- Never put on any hat over wet hair; the dryer the hair, the better the springback when you remove the hat.

- After removing your hat, switch your part to the opposite side: It gives instant fullness on top.

- After removing your hat, bend over, shake your head, then fluff up the hair from underneath. Or bend your head and brush downward a few times.

- Wear earmuffs instead of a hat.

Thirteen-year-old Anna, from Cedar City, Utah, is usually a gym nut in pigtails, but you'd never know it when she's transformed into a stunner in a black velvet jacket, simple white shirt, and a pink satin tie over suede, jeans-style pants. That freshly ironed hair makes her look really cool.

You ask: I have thin hair and my ponytail hangs there, limper than a sick puppy's tail. What can I do to make it look thicker?

Vincent: I love this question. Start by lightly back-combing about an inch of hair behind each ear and a few strands more in the back. Pull the whole thing back and secure it with a covered elastic, keeping your ponytail low—not perked high. Put a little gel in your hands and smooth down any parts that stick out too much. Your ponytail will be thick and luxurious like, well, a pony's tail. Tuck a great gorgeous flower into the elastic or wrap interesting ribbon around it. Then pull a few tendrils of hair loose at the sides and let them frame your face. Pretty girl!

You ask: Humidity is my enemy; my hair absolutely drops dead from moisture in the air. Any hope, any help?

Vincent: Sure. It's a common problem for most teens because almost all kinds of hair lose shape from humidity. But, on humid days, if you apply a product containing silicone and moisturizer on your wet hair, like Mario Tricoci's *3P-1 Styling Cream,* then blow-dry your hair straight, you have a good chance of beating the devil.

You ask: So, how can I find a hairstylist who's good with teen hair?

Vincent: When you see girls with great hair on the street, stop them. I'm not kidding. Who wouldn't like to be told she looks so terrific you'd like to use her hairstylist? If you see someone about your age whose hair looks great, just approach her with a smile and say something like, "This is sooo embarrassing to ask, but could you tell me who does your hair—it's terrific!" If you simply can't do that, ask the same of your friends, cousins, classmates, or teammates with great hair.

Make sure you don't look your slobbiest when you see a new hairdresser; the way you dress and use makeup tells the hairstylist how you feel about yourself. And, if you haven't paid much attention to yourself, don't expect the stylist to give you her or his undivided attention.

When you get there, here are some ways to judge if you're going to be compatible with the hairstylist:

1. Does he or she take time for a consultation, even before your hair is shampooed? Does the stylist pay attention to any photographs you may have brought that illustrate the hairstyle you want?

2. Does she or he ask about your shampoo and styling habits and how much time you want to spend on your hair daily?

3. Does he or she concentrate completely on you during the cut and styling, even if Sarah Hughes is sitting in the next chair?

You ask: I have a perspiration problem. What can I do?

Vincent: Probably your parents had the same problem. How much you perspire is controlled by your genes. Wear natural fibers like cotton and light wools that breathe—allow air to get between your clothes and your body. Try an antiperspirant/deodorant that controls wetness and odor (just a deodorant doesn't do it). If nothing works, your doctor can prescribe a stronger antiperspirant.

You ask: I have a mustache and I'm dying of embarrassment. What do I do?

Vincent: Try *Surgi-Cream,* a great depilatory, which removes hair by dissolving it at the skin's surface, providing a clean look that lasts for about a week before regrowth is visible. If you just want to lighten the hair, try Jolen *Cream Bleach*. The result can last for about three weeks. Waxing pulls the hair out at the follicle, and the area will be hairless for about a month, but all that pulling-out *smarts*! Tweezing is not a good idea for mustache hairs: It's very irritating to a sensitive area. Never shave facial hair—the growing-back stubble looks terrible! If the hair is really hard to remove or hide, consider having it removed in a salon by a professional electrolysist. In this country, mustaches on girls are definitely not cool.

You ask: When is the best time to pop a pimple?

Vincent: The best time? Never.

You add: C'mon, Vincent—be realistic. You want me to go to a major party with a tornado pimple about to blast off?

Vincent: Okay, okay. Try a warm compress on the site, then take a hot shower, and see if the pimple drains by itself. You can make a monster out of the volcano by squeezing the pimple and instead of pushing the guck out, you push it in and make it triple terrible. See page 123 for more advice on emergency zit treatment.

You ask: Yikes—I'm losing my hair faster than my dad's losing his. Am I doomed?

Vincent: Stop freaking and listen to Uncle Vincent. It's perfectly normal to shed from fifty to a hundred hairs a day (and even more during the spring and fall). It may also be that your hair is too brittle and is breaking off mid-hair, but that's very different from losing it from the scalp, like your dad does. You probably could use more conditioning. Avoid chemical color and too much heat from your blow-dryer. Also, try massaging your scalp to increase the blood flow necessary for hair strength and growth. Throw all those tight, uncovered rubber bands you use on your ponytail out the window. And when you remove even covered elastics, barrettes, clips, hair additions, and other accessories from your hair, do it gently. No yanking allowed.

You ask: How can I get makeup to last more than an hour or so?

Vincent: Start with a layer of oil-free moisturizer to give the makeup something to stick to. Finish with a powder puff (instead of a brush) of loose powder.

You ask: Getting dumped by a boyfriend hurts more than anything else in the world. It happened. Any suggestions on how to cope?

Vincent: You're right—it's a bummer. But *hair revenge* is the best defense. Choose a new style, reinvent yourself. Look so cool, he'll eat his heart out. (See page 93 for the *I-got-dumped* haircut.)

You ask: How do you know when you look cool?

Vincent: Easy. Check out the following cool list:

- *Presence*. Do you walk tall even if you're short? Do you act confident even when you're not? Do others hang on your words? You're cool.

- *Hair*. Is it healthy? Is it "swingy"? Is it interesting or pretty or both? You're cool.

- *Makeup and skin*. Is it subtle-natural by day, glam by moonlight, *clean* looking? You're cool.

- *Clothes*. Do you have personal style instead of being a slave to trendiness—the latest fad? You're cool.

- *Accessories*. Do you follow the *less-is-more* rule? In other words, do you wear just enough interesting jewelry to make a statement, not write a book? Do you wear one scarf—not three? You're cool.

- *A great book*. Do you always have reading material close by? Cool teens are generally good readers. Tucked into their purse or back-pack is a novel, book of poetry, or even a classy magazine—great for starting a conversation. If you're almost never without an interesting read within reach, you're cool.

You ask: I have a cowlick that stands right up at my hairline. What can I do to tame it?

Vincent: Easy. Use a blow-dryer or a tiny roller to teach the cowlick to blend into your hairstyle. A good gel works wonders and so does a product like Mario Tricoci's *Paste,* which molds the hair into the direction you want it to go.

You ask: My best friend talks about me behind my back. Do I give her up for dead?

Vincent: Well, it depends on what she's saying. Many of us talk about people we love behind their backs—and we're not being mean or disloyal.

Haven't you ever talked about your mom, your sister, or *your* best friend? Even when we love someone, sometimes we have to let off steam about her—especially when she irritates us. But if you hear that your best friend is telling your secrets or saying very nasty things that could ruin your reputation, that's not cool at all. That's simply rude and crude and disloyal. So don't give her up for dead, unless she's been saying unforgivable things. Simply confront her with what you know—and talk it out.

You ask: I keep having the same hair emergency. On a humid day, my hair frizzes up wildly. Soon, I have a job interview. What if it's humid out?

Vincent: Rub some hair gel between your hands (I like Bain de Terre's *Currant Expressions*) and slick down that dampened hair behind your ears. Or pull the gelled hair back in a ponytail or neat bun. These are great, no-nonsense, and very stylish looks for short and long hair—especially in an emergency.

You ask: I did it—shaved my arms right before the prom. I couldn't help it—they were too hairy! This is a hair emergency of a different kind because now my mom tells me the hair's going to grow back all stubbly. Is she right?

Vincent: Probably. You've shaved off the soft, tapered end of your arm hair. But don't panic. Wear long sleeves and in about a month, the hair will start getting soft and tapered again. Next time, either use a depilatory or go to a salon and have them wax your arms; this pulls the hair out at the root, which means no stubble.

You ask: My hair's suddenly gone frizzy and I can hardly style it. What gives?

Vincent: You've probably damaged it with too much brushing, bleaching, or coloring. Try this experiment: Pluck out about six or seven hairs, drop them in a glass of water, and tap them with your finger a couple of times. Do they sink or float? If they float, your hair's not damaged. Perhaps you need a better, more layered haircut—one you can easily blow-dry with a fat, round brush. If the hairs sink, they're absorbing moisture—a sign of some damage. Try a very deep protein conditioning treatment weekly. The protein molecules fill in the open pores of your hair, strengthening it.

You ask: My mom and dad are so strict. I want to have fun with my hair, but if I even mention a blue hair extension, they hit the ceiling. How can I assure them that I'll always be the same me—even with temporarily blue hair?

Vincent: It's hard. I had the same anxiety about my own daughter, Dawn. What worked for me was lots of reassurance from her that she would always be careful. She reminded me that hair was always a safe place to experiment because it would grow back.

And she was right.

Epilogue

To all my young clients as well as the teenagers I've never met: I think you are extraordinary young women, coming of age in difficult times. I'm immensely grateful for your confidence and for allowing me into your complicated lives.

I never thought that being a teenager was easy. I can remember that many of the most exciting moments in my life happened before I was twenty—like falling in love and starting an incredible career—but some of the most awkward and difficult moments also came during my teen years. For me, they were the years when passion and promise but also worry were strongest. I worried about everything—would I make it in the big world? Would I be attractive to others? Teenagers, and I was no exception, feel everything so powerfully.

I may not know you personally, but I can tell you this: You have the potential for all-around cool, not just cool hair. The way you wear your hair, dress, speak, think, present yourself are a package—a package of an *interesting young woman*. This doesn't mean that you can't regularly change the way you wear your hair, dress, speak, think, and present yourself. I'd be disappointed if you stayed the same. That's what makes you interesting.

But somehow, the essence of cool stays the same throughout your incarnations. A cool girl is, well, just cool. She likes herself and that allows her to open to others. She can tell her deepest secrets to people she trusts. Her comfort level is high. She feels that she looks her very best and is worthy of loving and being loved. You'll know her when you see her. You'll know her when you *are* her.

Here's what I want to say to you: When the world seems crazy, when life seems dark and very serious, when it's tough to keep your self-esteem high—I'd like you to think of the artist Cyndi Lauper and her earliest theme, *"Girls

Just Want to Have Fun." Of course, there's a lot more you want besides fun, but, whenever possible, do let the lighthearted, self-affirming part of yourself soar free. How?

In my book, the best way to have fun is to experiment with your look. Actually, most girls have been in training to be teens ever since they've been two— right? Remember getting into your mom's makeup and hair spray, your big sister's new sweatpants when you were in grade school?

So now that you're really there, go with it! Cool hair, cool makeup, and most of all cool attitude gladden the heart and raise the spirit like nothing else. Seize the moment.

Come see me in my salon! We'll talk cool.

Teens in training: Rebecca Goldstein, 12; Sienna Danielle Amato, 2; Julia Cohen, 7.
(Sienna's clothes by Burberry.)

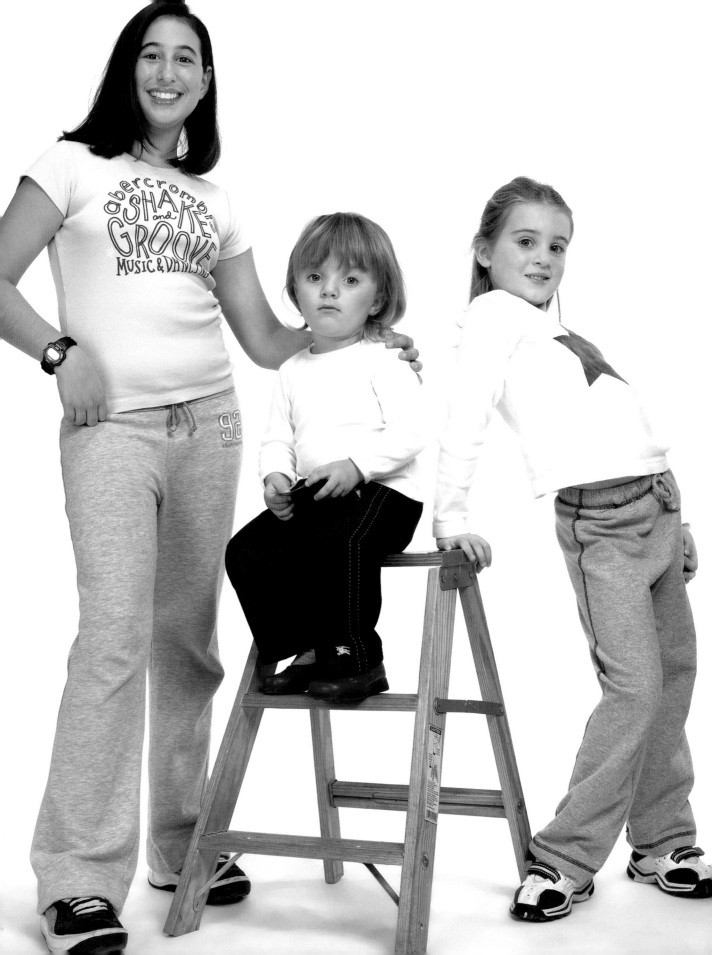

Acknowledgments

The idea for *Cool Hair* came from our inspired, beautiful, and incredibly cool editor, Diane Reverand. She's a legend in the world of publishing, but she's never forgotten how it feels to be eighteen. Alex Cao, our deeply talented and indisputably *hot* photographer, was the backbone for *Cool Hair.* We had marvelous fun at his studio, and this book owes so much to his magical artist's eye. Alex's team—Hiroki Sakamoto, Arlene Caballero, and D. Tyler Huff—were always helpful. We appreciate them!

The wonderful drawings are from Wendy DeFeudis (www.verywendy.com). She's an imaginative artist and fashion designer and will do custom designs and illustrations for your party invitations, clothing, or perhaps *your* book.

Thanks to Mel Berger of the William Morris Literary Agency, a great agent and, more important, father of Molly.

Cynthia Strickland, the beautiful and gentle director of Saks's *One on One* personal shopping service, made the *Cool Hair* looks come alive with the wonderful clothes she chose for our models from incomparable Saks Fifth Avenue. Almost every large department store has a shopping service for individuals seeking fashion advice—and it's usually free.

A real thank-you to Janet Denyer of the incredible Elizabeth Arden Red Door Salon for her inspired help. Daisy Chin was also wonderful.

Many of the makeup and hairstyling products were used courtesy of Elizabeth Arden; and Adriana Lima, a makeup artist for Elizabeth Arden Red Door Salon, provided us with useful information. Daisy Bailey, a makeup artist and skin specialist for Elizabeth Arden Red Door Salon, was extraordinarily helpful in rounding up products for our shoots. Angela Portella was terrific.

Deborah Wynns, Marilyn Sanchez, and Gise Lee—Vincent's magnificently talented hair staff—gave their all at every shoot. Natalie Marshall, Vincent's personal assistant, pulled it all together with her calm and steady self and stopped for only a moment to have a baby boy. Cecelia Brown, of the Elizabeth Arden Salon, was helpful and always smiling.

Kaori Kobayashi is the makeup artist for Uslu Airlines (a great makeup tool, not an airplane), and her delicate and exquisite work is featured in this book. Melanie L. Swanson, Jonnie Buick of Tiffany Whitford, Sacha Harford, and Elisa Flowers from Bernstein and Andriulli are also talented makeup artists who shared their expertise with our teenage models.

The wonderful young women who allowed us to photograph them for this book are stars—every one of them! We're particularly grateful to Eva Amurri, Pamela Brown, Jennifer Coleman, Lindsay Lohan, Lindsay Anderson, and the extraordinary Sarah Hughes.

Always love and gratitude to Vincent's two loyal pals—the most fabulous blondes in town, Diane Sawyer and Liz Smith.

We are enormously indebted to Saks Fifth Avenue—Vincent's home—for the exquisite fashions and many beauty and skin care products. This marvelous place is the quintessential specialty store—they don't make 'em like this anymore. And Chris Fields of Saks is unique.

Thanks also to Rebecca Goldstein and Julia Cohen for their knowing words on what's in and what's out and to Josh and Ben Goldstein and Peter Cohen for being the cutest guys in America.

Such love to our cool, patient families: Jude Roppatte; Dawn, Tony, and Sienna Amato; Larry Cohen; Jennifer and Steven Goldstein; Susan Gross and Adam Cohen.

Thanks to Beth Teitelman from the 92 Street Y who, in telling about her own teenager, first introduced the concept of hair being a *safe* place to experiment—far better than drugs or early sex.

Janet Hill Prystowsky, M.D., the very wise New York dermatologist, set us straight on skin.

We are immensely grateful to Jimi Mastrangelo of Ray's Beauty Supply Company in New York City for the wonderful hair ornaments and beauty supplies.

St. Martin's cool people—the incomparable Melissa Contreras, Nicole Liebowitz, and Steve Snider. Gisela Ramos worked tirelessly to make sure our book reaches the best people in the best magazines.

Our heartfelt gratitude to David Stoup, chairman and CEO of Trilogy Ventures, an extraordinary man who supported this book with friendship and warmth. David—you're the best. Also, the best looking. Finally and always, love and gratitude for Connie Clausen.